MEDICAL HUMANITIES

This ground-breaking book sets out a fresh vision for a future medical education by providing a radical reconceptualisation of the purposes of medical humanities through a lens of critical health psychology and liberatory pedagogy. The medical humanities are conceived as translational media through which reductive, instrumental biomedicine can be raised in quality, intensity, and complexity by embracing ethical, aesthetic, political, and transcendental values. This translation occurs through innovative use of metaphor. A note of caution is offered – that the medical humanities too can be instrumental and reductive if not framed well.

Drawing on major theorists such as Michel Foucault and Jacques Rancière and bringing together insights from diverse but inter-related fields, Bleakley focuses on the "ills" of contemporary biomedicine and medical education, and the need for reconceptualisation, which – it is argued – the translational medical humanities have the potential to accomplish. Current instrumental approaches to medical humanities, embracing communication skills training and narrative-based medicine, have failed to address the chronic symptoms suffered by medicine. These include resort to closed, functional systems thinking rather than embracing dynamic, complex, open, and adaptive systems thinking; lack of democratic habits in medical culture, compromising patient safety and care; the production of insensibility rather than deepening of sensibility in medical education; a lack of attention to ethics, aesthetics, and politics where the instrumental is privileged; and a lack of critical reflexivity in revisioning habitual practices. Through persuasive argument, Bleakley sets out a more radical manifesto for the role the arts and humanities might play in medical/healthcare education and offers a new approach based on curriculum process rather than syllabus content, to recuperate aesthetic sensibilities, discernment, and affect in medicine.

The book will appeal to medical and healthcare educators, medical and health humanities scholars, engaged clinicians, social scientists drawing on critical theory, and arts and humanities practitioners engaging with medical and healthcare themes.

Dr Alan Bleakley is Emeritus Professor of Medical Education and Medical Humanities at Plymouth University Peninsula Medical School, UK. He is past President of the Association of Medical Humanities.

Critical Approaches to Health

Series Editors: Kerry Chamberlain & Antonia Lyons

The Routledge *Critical Approaches to Health* series aims to present critical, interdisciplinary books around psychological, social and cultural issues related to health. Each volume in the series provides a critical approach to a particular issue or important topic, and is of interest and relevance to students and practitioners across the social sciences. The series is produced in association with the International Society of Critical Health Psychology (ISCHP).

Titles in the series:

Embodied Trauma and Healing
Critical Conversations on the Concept of Health
Anna Westin

Migration and Health
Critical Perspectives
Heide Castañeda

Rethinking Global Health
Frameworks of Power
Rochelle A. Burgess

Medical Humanities
Ethics, Aesthetics, Politics
Alan Bleakley

For more information about this series, please visit: https://www.routledge.com/Critical-Approaches-to-Health/book-series/CRITHEA

MEDICAL HUMANITIES

Ethics, Aesthetics, Politics

Alan Bleakley

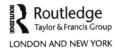

Routledge
Taylor & Francis Group

LONDON AND NEW YORK

Designed cover image: Getty Images

First published 2024
by Routledge
4 Park Square, Milton Park, Abingdon, Oxon OX14 4RN

and by Routledge
605 Third Avenue, New York, NY 10158

Routledge is an imprint of the Taylor & Francis Group, an informa business

British Library Cataloguing-in-Publication Data
A catalogue record for this book is available from the British Library

ISBN: 9781032467856 (hbk)
ISBN: 9781032467849 (pbk)
ISBN: 9781003383260 (ebk)

DOI: 10.4324/9781003383260

Typeset in Times New Roman
by codeMantra

To my wife Sue for unstinting support, and to my family for their cradle of love and affection.

CONTENTS

FIGURES

ACKNOWLEDGEMENTS

I am grateful to the following colleagues.

Chapter 6 is adapted from a previous collaboration with Professor Jennifer Cleland; segments of Chapter 8 from a previous collaboration with Professor Margaretta Jolly; and Chapters 9 and 10 result from a longstanding collaboration with Dr Shane Neilson.

I am grateful to Dr Robert Marshall for collaborative support, especially during the heyday of Peninsula Medical School's medical humanities innovations.

I would like to thank Kerry Chamberlain, Antonia Lyons, and Lucy Kennedy for setting this book in motion, and Lakshay Gaba for completing the cycle.

SERIES EDITORS' PREFACE

Critical approaches to health

Health is a major issue for people all around the world, and is fundamental to individual wellbeing, personal achievements, and satisfaction, as well as to families, communities, and societies. It is also embedded in social notions of participation and citizenship. Much has been written about health, from a variety of perspectives and disciplines, but a lot of this writing takes a biomedical and positivist approach to health matters, neglecting the historical, social, and cultural contexts and environments within which health is experienced, understood, and practiced. It is timely for a new series of books that offer critical, social science perspectives on important health topics.

The *Critical Approaches to Health* series provides new writing on health by presenting books offering critical, interdisciplinary, and theoretical writing about health, where matters of health are framed quite broadly. The series seeks to include books that range across important health matters, including general health-related issues (such as gender and media), major social issues for health (such as medicalisation, obesity, and palliative care), particular health concerns (such as pain, doctor-patient interaction, health services, and health technologies), particular health problems (such as diabetes, autoimmune disease, and medically unexplained illness), or health for specific groups of people (such as the health of migrants, the homeless, and the aged), or combinations of these.

The series seeks above all to promote critical thought about health matters. By critical, we mean going beyond the critique of the topic and work in the field, to more general considerations of power and benefit, and in particular, to addressing concerns about whose understandings and interests are upheld and whose are marginalised by the approaches, findings, and practices in these various domains of health. Such critical agendas involve reflections on what constitutes knowledge, how it is created, and how it is used. Accordingly, critical approaches consider epistemological and theoretical positioning, as well as issues of methodology and practice, and seek to examine how health is enmeshed within broader social relations and structures. Books within this series take up this challenge and seek to provide new insights and understandings by applying a critical agenda to their topics.

In this book, *Medical Humanities: Ethics, Aesthetics, Politics*, Alan Bleakley considers the place of medical humanities in medicine. He describes how this field became established and how it has been marginalised and ignored within medicine, forcefully arguing that it can contribute substantially to medical education and care. If you have ever wondered whether the humanities can influence, change, and improve medicine, this book will leave you in no doubt. Within myriad critical discussions on the problems and limitations of medicine, medical training, and medical practice, the book offers a compelling case for why and how the inclusion of the humanities into medical education can increase the competencies of practitioners, the care which patients might receive, and the wellbeing of people working within the medical realm.

The core premise of the book is that medicine needs to shift from being dominated by systems thinking with values focussed on reductionism and instrumentalism, and move towards embracing aesthetic, ethical, political, and transcendental values. Bleakley offers a convincing argument for the medical humanities as the way to facilitate this transition, moving medicine from simple linear to more complex non-linear systems thinking – a move from positions of certainty to positions of uncertainty and ambiguity. This is necessary, he argues, because medicine itself is overly conservative and resistant to innovation, and because the work of healthcare is necessarily complex and nonlinear in most of its endeavours, frequently working "at the edge of chaos". Engaging medicine with medical humanities, Bleakley suggests, can shift the register of medicine to increase its potential to tolerate ambiguity, and in this way improve both practice and care.

Providing an alternative translational approach to medicine, the book provides a detailed and critical account that offers nuanced ways in which medicine and medical education can be improved. It is holistic in that it shows how patients can be involved in medical education, and how medical care can advance if more attention was given to medical humanities and to humanities in general. This would enhance medicine, medical education, and the medical encounter. This book is wide-ranging in coverage, full of innovative ideas, critical analyses, and aspirational directions, all in the service of changing the register of medical science in partnership with the medical humanities, and transforming instrumental and economic biomedicine into an aesthetic, ethical, political, and spiritual practice.

Medical Humanities: Ethics, Aesthetics, Politics provides another important and apposite addition to the *Critical Approaches to Health* series, offering informative and challenging content, with compelling salience for contemporary medical education and practice.

Kerry Chamberlain & Antonia Lyons
March 2023

INTRODUCTION

The medical humanities: the art of productively increasing the metaphor count

Deep in the bowels of academia there is a room with a single desk and chair and the door is shut tight. Here, a neuroscientist sits, fervently believing that the joys and tragedies of life – joyous lovemaking, bringing up children, forming a government, engaging in climate activism – can be explained by the firing of neurons in particular parts of the brain. While this explanation may be complex within its own limited domain, it is reductive in stripping away all other contexts for explanation – personal, social, cultural, historical, and ecological. More, driven mainly by an instrumental value complex, this explanation may also strip away other values shaping human experience such as the ethical, aesthetic, political, and spiritual.

In a book about the frontiers of cell biology, the oncologist Siddhartha Mukherjee (2022) explores how he fell into a deep depression where he was "drowning in a tide of sadness I could not swim past or through". As a cell biologist, Mukherjee's clinical and academic world, like that of the imagined neuroscientist above, promises a reductive perspective. For his cancer patients, his primary focus and explanatory level is cellular, where such cells divide and rage out of control. So, as the atmosphere of depression descends upon Mukherjee's being, "it was only natural that I would try to understand the core of my depression in terms of abnormalities in neurons in my brain". Yet, here is the cell biologist and physician drawing on swimming and drowning metaphors to describe his depression: "a tide of sadness".

On his exploratory journey, Mukherjee meets up with the Nobel prize-winning neuroscientist Paul Greengard, who explains that Mukherjee may have a "slow brain problem". Another metaphor. Communication between neurons through chemical neurotransmitters is normally rapid (we're talking milliseconds), where "slow" transmission between synapses can take seconds, even minutes. More, across complex brain circuits, "slow" transmission may take days. This is called a "slow cascade". Depression, says Greengard, is a "flaw" in cells, in neurons and

DOI: 10.4324/9781003383260-1

in neurotransmission. All of this affects overall levels of serotonin in the brain, thought to affect mood. But, says Greengard, it is not just the level of serotonin, but rather how the serotonin acts on the individual neuron at a cellular level that causes depressive episodes.

Mukherjee is wise enough in this book to recognise the value of metaphor. Indeed, see how the metaphors have already piled up ("slow brain problem", "slow cascade"), elevating the instrumental understanding of neuronal activity to a higher level of meaning. This is not simply a burnishing, but a truly significant leap – jumping a metaphorical synapse.

Mukherjee (ibid.: 291–96) describes the work of Helen Mayberg, a neurologist, who is experimenting with electrical stimulation of specific deep areas of the brain that may be linked to depressive episodes – a therapy aimed at adjusting brain circuits through direct intervention. Patients that Mayberg has treated this way also describe their depressions through metaphors such as: "trapped inside a hole, a void", "stuck in a cave", and "pushed down by force fields". Talking to Mukherjee, Mayberg says: "I hadn't realised it then, but listening to the metaphors was absolutely vital. It was the metaphors that allowed me to track whether a patient was responding or not" (to the deep electro-stimulation treatment). On stimulation, one patient said: "the void lifted", and reported seeing herself "lifted out of the sinkhole and sitting on a rock … above the hole". So, for this person, is it the deep brain stimulation *and* the metaphor that heals or relieves suffering? Well yes, the metaphor is essential because *metaphor creates meaning where previously meaning was absent*. Previously, there was just information. Information alone can of course cure, but meaning introduces care.

Of course, the little room (above) where our neuroscientist sits is also a metaphor – for a "cell", the smallest whole biological unit. The word was coined by the English scientist Robert Hooke for what he saw under the newly invented microscope, from the Latin *cella* for "small room", the root also of "cellar" and a prison or religious retreat "cell". But, when lips touch, skin on skin, in a passionate kiss, do you immediately think of neurons firing or animated cells? No, you enjoy the bigger sensation and cherish the emotions. Of course, your neurons are firing and so are your partner's, but your experience is bigger, more expansive, embracing. You are on a beach, the full moon is out, there is a warm breeze and a distinctive smell of sea air, while your touch is at first tentative. You are embraced by a context. Immanuel Kant thought that "reality" was all in the head, while the neuroscientists force us even deeper inward, away from the reality of the tang of that sea air and the way that skin on skin feels in careful, intimate, and sensual encounters.

Of course, if neurons were not firing then we wouldn't be experiencing at all. But while we do, the experience surely cannot be reduced just to brain activity. Going down into the cellular level generally can, of course, engage a cosmos. Just because we choose neuronal firings rather than social collectives as our unit of analysis does not mean that we must succumb to reductionism or functionalism. The key here is that complex systems work at all levels of nature, from the global (such as weather systems) to the local (such as DNA building proteins) (see Chapter 6). This is the world of fractals (another metaphor) – structures, forms and patterns repeating themselves at different levels of size. But, as we move from, say, a social grouping to a neuron firing, a cell dividing, and the chemistry of serotonin, there is a tendency to frame form in terms of function. Then we reduce the metaphorical "chemistry" of the kiss to a literal chemistry and biology of epidermis on epidermis.

While Greengard and Mayberg above, channelled in Mukherjee's fascinating book, drive us into the basement room in which the lonely neuroscientist sits with the door closed, again they make sense of (or bring into the sensory world) their interests through metaphor: "slow cascade" and "sinkholes". Switching attention to the meanings and purposes of those metaphors, our lonely and isolated neuroscientist opens the door of her room and, despite being in the basement, light comes flooding in. She steps out from a world insistent on the value of quantities into the world of qualities. Here, she reads Mukherjee's book under an apple tree in the university's gardens, and in so doing ratchets up her experience to enjoy metaphorical showers of language about brain science. An apple falls. In Newtonian wonder, a whole new world of values emerges. While bioscience models of neuronal firing or cellular activity may inform understanding, it does not explain experience. For this, we need a wider spectrum of approaches drawn from the arts and humanities.

This step into wider existence does not deny the immense value of the information gleaned from reductive neuroscience. Rather, it reminds us that neuroscience can be nourished and expanded where it shifts away from its base in utility and function to embrace aesthetic (beauty, form), ethical (justice), political (power), and spiritual (transcendental) concerns. Enter the medical humanities in medicine and medical education, where the primary function of this eclectic range of approaches drawn from the arts, humanities and qualitative social sciences is to raise the aspirations of biomedical science from the instrumental to embrace a spectrum of values and qualities. Biomedical science's potential is realised as it engages with other disciplinary forms such as the arts and humanities in processes of translation.

Having worked in the field of medical humanities internationally over many years, I can say without hesitation that many medical humanities advocates, even from within medicine, seem oblivious to the value of working the medical humanities from the base of biomedical sciences out, facilitating the recovery of biomedical science's potential as an approach of beauty and quality. Rather, science and art get into an unnecessary tussle, reflecting a longstanding and unfortunate opposition. The medical humanities are then invoked as supposed compensation for science's perceived lack. But, without diluting the power of the arts and humanities to add important voices to medical and healthcare debates, what if we were to concentrate on releasing biomedical science from the longstanding grip of reductionist values to allow it to express its worth through a range of values?

This book offers an overview of current trends in the medical humanities, including both key distinctions and points of intersection between the medical and health humanities. The medical humanities are further distinguished axiologically as two distinct fields. The first – medical humanities in medical education – is largely pedagogically oriented, aiming to improve the undergraduate education of medical students (Bleakley 2015) and postgraduate or continuing education of doctors (Peterkin and Skorzewska 2018). This is embedded in the larger aim to improve patient care and safety. The second – medical culture as a topic for interdisciplinary study – deals with how biomedicine is legitimated, represented, and expressed as viewed through arts and humanities lenses (Whitehead and Woods 2016).

The "medical humanities" are used in the plural to describe a complex of approaches drawn from the arts, humanities and qualitative social sciences focused on generating, expanding, and investigating qualities, rather than quantities, in medicine. They are grounded in a simple mantra: appreciation before explanation. As noted, a distinction is drawn between the medical humanities and the growing field of the "health humanities" (Crawford, Brown and Charise 2020). This more inclusive term has, for some, superseded the "medical humanities" (Jones, Wear and Friedman 2014). But I argue that it is important to maintain key distinctions between these two, as differing Bourdieuian "fields". The medical humanities focus upon:

i use of the arts, humanities, and qualitative social sciences in *medical* education to improve patient care and safety (based largely in *medical* schools); and
ii the academic, critical study of *medical* culture (based largely in university departments).

In contrast, the health humanities focus upon:

i the use of arts and humanities across the health- and social-care education and practice spectrums;
ii the academic study of wider health- and social-care; and
iii uncritical use of the "available arts" for therapeutic purposes through public participation.

I offer a critical reading of current developments and provocations in the field of the medical humanities, articulating a new perspective. My focus is upon medical humanities in medical education as this aligns with current developments in curriculum reconceptualisation pedagogy (Pinar 2019). The spirit of the book rests with extending the question "what are the medical humanities?" to "what is possible within the field of medical humanities?" The first question remains descriptive, where the second is exploratory.

This book is written from the point of view of critical health psychology and liberatory pedagogy as these interact with key medical humanities traditions and developments. I argue that the medical humanities can be situated to offer a form of "sly civility" resistance (Bhabha 2004) to a dominant discourse of biomedicine characterised by functionalism and instrumentalism. "Sly civility" is a sophisticated, knowing form of resistance to an oppressive dominant discourse that draws on Thoreau's and Ghandi's "civil disobedience" and Franz Fanon's "combat breathing" (Bleakley 2020a). But this approach does not simply reject biomedicine for its instrumentalism. In fact, just the opposite – it is restorative. *In the process, and surprisingly, this act of resistance uncovers an aesthetically, ethically, politically, and spiritually sensitive biomedicine that has been inhibited through formal medical education.* Arguing that a traditional medical education is to some extent a "compulsory mis-education" (Goodman 1966) based on production of insensibility (Bleakley 2020b), once such inhibitions are articulated and lifted, medicine can flourish. "Critical" is taken as a political, ethical, and aesthetic gesture that inquires below the surface of representations to reveal deeper sources and motivations for such surface phenomena. This imbues the medical humanities with a hermeneutics of suspicion – that what medicine and medical education preach is not always what they practice, and that what is practiced is sometimes deeply unaware of its flaws and fault-lines. I take as a starting point that medicine and medical education display symptoms and need to be treated (see Chapters 4 and 5). Within a psychoanalytic frame, this constitutes a revelation of what is repressed and has returned in a distorted form. Here, the medical humanities play a key therapeutic role.

The medical humanities in clinical practice and medical education can be defined as *the art of productively increasing the metaphor count.* This is, of course, the everyday work of the arts, humanities, and qualitative social sciences in general, from improvised jazz, radical performance art, audience-led theatre, innovative visual art, expressive dance, and critical studies, to feminist critique, liberatory pedagogies, mad studies, and good qualitative social science research. As the metaphor count rises, so the public body is "healthier" in the sense of increasing intensity, quality, and complexity of life. In other words: generating meaning from mere information, putting form before function, and seeking non-invasive connection with the natural world.

1

BORN IN THE USA

Origin myths of the medical humanities

Serendipity

It was June 2021, just after a UK-wide Covid lockdown had been lifted. My wife had a few days' work in the wilds of mid-Wales, and I had some research to do on a book manuscript. We had booked to stay at a small boutique hotel tucked away in the countryside, miles from urban life. We arrived at the hotel, which was lavishly decorated with beautiful antiques and paintings. The co-owner showed us around. In welcome surprise, even slight shock, I recognised two paintings by the British painter Adrian Hill. I shared that I was researching Hill's work as part of a forth-coming book, and that this was fortunate coincidence on a large scale. The father of the man who was now showing me Hill's paintings had been a well-known and highly respected anaesthetist. The father had expected the son, my host, to follow him into medicine as a career. But instead, the son had developed a passion for racing vintage cars, that he now collected, and eschewed the far more prestigious profession of medicine. He explained that his father, the distinguished anaesthe-tist, had met Hill in the sanatorium where the painter was being treated, and sub-sequently they developed a close friendship. Hill had used drawing and painting therapeutically with other inmates in the sanatorium, facilitating their recoveries. He christened this work "art therapy", effectively laying the groundwork for the later development of both the medical and health humanities (Hill 1945). In all, there were over a dozen of Hill's works either displayed or stored at the hotel. Here, again, was a moment of deep serendipity – a fortunate coincidence.

"Serendipity" was the word coined by Horace Walpole in 1754 to describe the life courses of his heroes in *The Three Princes of Serendip* who "were always mak-ing discoveries, by accidents and sagacity, of things they were not in quest of". "Serendip" referred to Ceylon, now Sri Lanka. Serendipity was then configured

DOI: 10.4324/9781003383260-2

by Walpole as mysterious, an aspect of Eastern inscrutability, and an 18th-century scratch-card – mostly you are unlucky, but sometimes you strike gold. We would now see this association between mystery and the "inscrutable East" as a blatant Western, colonial, "Orientalist" projection (Said 1978). But the abstract idea of serendipity, or fortunate chance, is a good one – readily advertised in, for example, Isaac Newton observing the apple falling from the tree, subject to what would come be termed "gravity". Indeed, isn't life itself, consciousness, a product of serendipity? Evolution by natural selection is, after all, the product of chance mutations in genes.

Adrian Hill was the official war artist during the 1914–18 Great War and continued to pursue a career as a successful painter. In 1944, he contracted tuberculosis and was admitted to a sanatorium for recovery. In *Art Versus Illness,* published in 1945, Hill describes how he began to draw and paint to help his recuperation. (After our visit to Wales, I managed to track down a copy of Hill's book, now quite rare. It remains a prized possession.) In Hill's work, marking the beginning of the art therapy movement in the UK as noted above, we also have an "origin myth" for the modern medical humanities. Although maybe we should give that honour to the mother of nursing, Florence Nightingale, who said in 1860:

> The effect in sickness of beautiful objects, of variety of objects, and especially of brilliancy of colours is hardly at all appreciated … People say the effect is only on the mind. It is no such thing. The effect is on the body too. … Variety of form and brilliancy of colour in the objects presented to patients is an actual means of recovery.

Drawing on inspiration such as that advertised by Nightingale above and encouraged by suggestions from medical staff at the sanatorium, Hill began to encourage and support other patients to draw and paint, noting tangible success in terms of their improvement (both physical and psychological). While patients in hospitals had previously, on occasions, been encouraged to engage in an ad hoc manner with crafts such as basket weaving – largely to reduce boredom – Hill devised a formal educational programme. He taught technique to the sanatorium patients with whom he worked, and many produced passable art works. The term "medical humanities" would be coined a few years later, in 1948, by a chemist and historian of science George Sarton (Bleakley 2015). But the use was casual, and the term remained stagnant. A more widely adopted, properly rationalised, "medical humanities" would not emerge until the 1970s.

North American interests might contest that Adrian Hill should be celebrated as the founder of the medical humanities (in 1944–45) through art therapy, where this accolade could readily be bestowed upon Margaret Naumberg, working at a psychiatric institute in New York State in 1941–47. She published a series of case studies from this work, where her art therapy interventions were grounded in both Freudian and Jungian psychoanalysis, a mix of personal and transpersonal, or symbolic, dynamics. She named her method "dynamically-oriented art therapy". Let's give Naumberg and Hill equal status as co-founders of art therapy and then, in essence, the mother and father of the medical humanities.

A note on method

In formulating the critical analysis of the medical and health humanities (distinctions between the two will be made clear below) that is the subject of this book, I retain a historical perspective. To know where the medical and health humanities come from is also to gain a perspective on their current meanings and purposes. But it is important also to approach such a history critically. "History" here is taken not as a listing of events chronologically, set in a vacuum. Rather, such re-telling of events has contexts and interconnections, where their recall is necessarily partial and biased. Here, I draw on the approach of Michel Foucault towards the history of social phenomena (in Foucault's case topics include classification schemes and typologies of the natural world, madness, the medical clinic, human sexuality, the modern subject, and truth-telling or ethical conduct).

Foucault's (1970) initial approach to historical understanding was an "archaeology" of knowledge, focused particularly upon how phenomena come to be ordered or classified. Here, the researcher digs deep into the archives to discover supposed "origins" of phenomena. Later, Foucault (1976, 1991, 2005, 2006) abandons this archaeological approach – of metaphorically digging for the truth – to embrace a geneaological approach. Here, a family tree of resemblances circumscribing a particular phenomenon is described that does not seek an origin point, but rather puts together a set of conditions of possibility for the emergence of a novel phenomenon (again, such as "madness", "the medical clinic", "human sexuality", and "the modern self"). Thus, for the emergence of "madness" we find, through the early modern to the Enlightenment periods in Europe, a convergence of factors: leprosy disappears leaving empty lazar houses ripe for the internment of a new kind of inmate – the "insane"; in tandem, city authorities start to "clean up" the streets by incarcerating vagrants, prostitutes, and single mothers who had previously adopted the street as home; and psychiatry enters a phase of intense identification and treatment of psychological disorders (such as "hysteria"), previously tolerated as idiosyncratic behaviours to be tolerated rather than forms of illness to be treated.

Here, I ask: what are the conditions of possibility for the emergence of the medical and health humanities? Margaret Naumburg's and Adrian Hill's art therapy experiments are key nodes in this web, genealogy, or family tree. Allow me to identify some other nodes.

A medical humanities culture emerges in North America

Beyond the Naumberg and Hill connections, other histories of the origins of the medical humanities point to E. E. Reinke's 1937 call for "leavening technical (medical) training with a liberal education" (Bleakley 2015). Reinke, a Professor of Biology at Vanderbilt University in Nashville, Tennessee, called specifically for the education of liberal values in premedical education, so that medical students would arrive at medical school with a rounded, humanistic education. There was a long tradition of medicine's relationship to literature and music for example, and doctors would be expected to have an education in the Classics. But by the 1930s, as Reinke notes, medicine was in the grip of a scientific revolution where biomedical inquiry was already clouding traditions of bedside manner so that patients became objectified, seen for their symptoms alone. Reinke's call was followed in 1948 by the first known use of the term "medical humanities" in print. As noted earlier, the Belgian-born American historian of science George Sarton used the term in a book review of, and obituary for, a linguist and historian where, "His death at the early age of 48 is a sad blow to the medical humanities, for very much could have been expected of him". The term was almost certainly used by Sarton to refer to his lifelong passion of bridging the sciences and humanities. While the term "medical humanities" was not further developed by Sarton, it seems to be coined with much confidence, as if it were already in circulation to describe how the gaze of humanities scholars could be directed towards medical culture.

Two key foundation stones for the development of the medical humanities in North America were laid a decade apart. In an innovative curriculum overhaul between 1952 and 1957, Case Western Reserve medical school in Cleveland, Ohio introduced an optional medical history programme. In 1967, a curriculum overhaul at Pennsylvania State University's College of Medicine led to a community-based curriculum with an emphasis upon ethics, spirituality, and social justice. (Ironically, over half a century later, Creighton University Medical School, a faith-based school based in Omaha, Nebraska and Phoenix, Arizona, set up what was claimed to be an innovative medical humanities programme, also based on ethics, spirituality, and social justice.) At Case Western Reserve, an expansive biopsychosocial model was introduced, against the grain of the development of reductive biomedical approaches elsewhere.

It was not until the early 1970s that the medical humanities gained a serious foothold in medical education in North America. This was through three main channels – the growth of bioethics and law as discrete disciplines (tolerated in medical education for their obvious applicability to medical studies, but also because of an alarming rise in the number of medical negligence lawsuits in North America); interest in the history and philosophy of medicine; and interest in literature and medicine as the early seeds of the narrative medicine movement. The latter offered a humane alternative to the formal, instrumental, quantitative, and reductive medical charts and records tracking patients' progress. The main condition of possibility for the emergence of the medical humanities rested with the explosion of a reductive or instrumental scientific medicine. A need was perceived for a "warm" humanist medicine to counter the aggressive development of a "cold", objective biomedicine led by emerging technologies.

Another way of looking at this, and this is surely the primary condition of possibility for the emergence of the medical and health humanities, is that biomedical science becomes a "runaway" condition as a dominant discourse *in its reductive, instrumental, or functional guise* (embracing not only baseline biomedicine but also economics – monetary costs - as a dominant frame for medical provision and conduct). Here, other values complex positions are squashed or side-lined – such as the aesthetic, ethical, political, and transcendental. In recognition of this, and under the banner of "bioethics" and "medical humanities", efforts were made by bioethicists, historians of science, and scholars of literature to expand the purview of biomedicine to embrace more qualities. There was a perceived need, for example, to cultivate both the theory and application of biomedical sciences artistically or aesthetically in the wake of interest in ethical issues, and the necessity of more creative economic modelling within a medical school's budget that naturally ran up against a variety of political interests. Thinking such bioscience humanely and democratically would follow. But, as noted, one constellation of academics would spearhead the growth of medical humanities in North America – literary scholars intent on developing a "narrative-based medicine".

A historical condition of possibility attracted literary scholars to medical schools based on a hunch. As literature departments in American universities started to focus on ever-more exclusive, or ring-fenced, disciplines and sub-disciplines, so literature scholars interested in inter-disciplinary and trans-disciplinary work (for example, fiction and autoethnography grounded in medical work) were frozen out of the universities, where some gravitated to medical schools with a promise that they might "humanise" a perceived functional bioscience bias. Some medical faculty, more adventurous or liberal-minded physicians, invited literature scholars frozen out of their own universities to initiate narrative-based medicine studies in the medical academy. Who could resist? Key figures such as Anne Hudson-Jones and Kathryn Montgomery Hunter took up the offer and became trailblazers for the emergent "medical humanities", promised as a multi-disciplinary curriculum offering within (mainly undergraduate) medical education.

Doctors and medical educators in the post-WWII years embraced a fast-developing technological medicine where the focus of interest was primarily on the scientific object or technology that helped the patient, rather than on the patient herself. Medicine became reductive and instrumentally focused as it became more powerful and autocratic. By the 1980s, the counterweight-to-bioscience medical humanities had made significant inroads into medical education – enough to generate scepticism about the supposed "humanising" of a blunt but powerful biomedicine. In 1987, J.D. Wassersug, a physician and medical humanities sceptic, argued that "real medical progress has not been made by humanitarians but by doctors equipped with microscopes, scalpels, dyes, catheters, rays, test tubes, and culture plates". But the opposition between object-led/objective science and the humanities proved to be more in Wassersug's mind – shaped by a tired oppositional model of arts vs sciences – than reality.

Wassersug's utterance will serve as a seed for the kind of critical thinking about the medical humanities that informs and shapes this book. While outwardly dismissive, Wassersug's very sentence here is, ironically, surprisingly poetic. The sceptic's barbed criticism disguises unacknowledged literary treasures. Let's look again at Wassersug's complaint: "real medical progress has not been made by humanitarians but by doctors equipped with microscopes, scalpels, dyes, catheters, rays, test tubes, and culture plates". It benefits from the hard "s" plural consonance. It has rhythm. And while all the objects listed are – in a functional worldview – instruments used instrumentally, they can also be read as both media for beauty and form, and for political machinations. So, these pieces of equipment glow and give off presence. They are animated artefacts as extensions of the flesh of persons who use them, such as surgeons. Everyday pieces of surgical equipment can be treated expansively and poetically rather than reductively and instrumentally: "grasping forceps", "skin hooks", "needle holders", "tapered needles", "locking forceps", "rake retractors". These become metaphors rather than literal descriptors in the eyes of somebody attuned to the aesthetic in medicine and surgery – albeit potentially "tough" metaphors, even bullying ("grasping", "hooks", "needle", "locking") (and then ironic within the field of surgery, known for its historical record of stiff hierarchies and blatant bullying). And here is a key point for the reconstructive medical humanities that engage a critical approach to health. We must move beyond the bottom line of the currently dominant instrumental and economic values to embrace more complex aesthetic, ethical, political, and transcendental approaches.

But what, precisely, is meant by the "medical humanities"?

In his rush to oppose humanities and science, and then to excise the humanities from the body of biomedicine, we can see that Wassersug's tactic backfires by failing to recognise the art and humanity already present in his "hard" science, particularly as a presence of metaphor that he cannot excise, and of which he appears to be ignorant. As noted, equipment such as surgical objects provide a ready-made poetics – albeit a "tough" one – in their physical designs; and a feast of metaphors in their linguistic descriptors: again, "grasping forceps", "skin hooks", "needle holders", "tapered needles", "locking forceps", "rake retractors", and so forth. Just rolling these descriptors in the mouth gives them presence and texture, and applying them in sentences introduces metaphorical thinking, rapidly expanding possibilities of language and sailing far away from the safe harbour of the instrumental or functional (including the base economic).

"Thinking with objects" is a key factor in both Plato's and Aristotle's view of *ekphrasis.* This is the expanded, vivid description of objects, often rhetorical, moving away from literalism to the metaphoric and then poetic. It is superbly advertised in John Keats' poetry – recalling that Keats abandoned a career in medicine and surgery for poetry – where objects attain an ontological status, or a state of being, equivalent to the person for whom the object is an extension of the senses (Harman 2018). Or object and person are identified in animation. Biomedicine can then be metaphor-rich and poetic rather than literal and mechanistic-reductive. Such technical medical language works against novel metaphor coinage and usage through standardisation and reduction to abstract terms. Thus, "dyspnea" is the medical term for "shortness of breath", but the physician-writer Jay Baruch (2022: 129) offers a better metaphor in the vernacular "air hunger". "Vomiting blood" becomes "haematemesis"; "panting for breath" "tachypnoea" (tak-ip-nee-uh); a black, tarry stool which is caused by upper gastrointestinal tract bleeding "melaena". Sometimes a historical, beautiful, elegant metaphor is reduced over time to a blunt and rather ugly instrumental term, such as "protoplasmic kisses" morphing into "synapses" – a literalism from the Greek *sunapsis* meaning "joining together" (Colón-Ramos 2016).

Again, these poetic descriptors can be tested from your armchair for the way in which they raise value or increase quality. Utter "panting for breath" and the phrase imitates the activity. The medico-scientific term "tachypnoea" has some chewy quality, but nothing like the hurried "panting-for-breath" in which the breath is literally panted in the saying. The technical term too is the capital of the medical professional and not of the patient, who owns the vernacular. Try saying "vomiting blood" – the speech imitates the act. It is embodied and has common ownership. The technical term "haematemesis" has a closed, professional ownership (which is fine – technical terms are useful) but doesn't bridge to patients and their felt symptoms in the same way that "vomiting blood" does, spectacularly. Do you see how the medical humanities can work? More, where the lay perception of medical humanities is probably about restoring humanity to medical encounters, here I am restoring vernacular descriptors of conditions to patients as a counter to medicine's literal (non-metaphorical) technical language.

But wait a minute, haven't I just said that "grasping forceps", "skin hooks", and so forth, are aesthetically interesting, yet these are technical terms? Yes, but this just adds to my argument. Usually, medico-technical terms are literal or non-metaphorical (of Greek or Roman origin) and in this sense "dead". These surgical equipment descriptors are rising from their linguistic graves not because surgeons are heralding their metaphoric worth, but because I am encouraging this line. Surgeons would probably rather stuff them back in their technical language containers.

Besides the aesthetic of medical equipment now being in plain view, such equipment is also inherently political where its design features advertise forms of power (such as "grasping", "locking", "retracting", and "hooking"). This is explicit in the scandals associated with the production of surgical equipment in sweatshops in Sialkot in Pakistan, sometimes drawing on child labour with evidence that such instruments have, historically, been in the English NHS supply chain (Randerson 2008; Tickle 2015).

Surgical equipment, for example, is a literal extension of a surgeon's persona and authority and as such has key semiotic importance. While surgical equipment is literally sterile (sterilised) it is semiotically fertile. Such equipment also affords labour for medicine. It is capital investment seeking profit. Procurement and use by more affluent medical services bring into sharp focus the differences in quality between high-income and lower-income countries' health economies. Sophisticated practical extensions to surgeons' hands and eyes, such as laparoscopic equipment, extend mechanics to aesthetics, for they are painterly and sculptural media. Such equipment predictably introduces economic, ethical, and political concerns to medicine; but primarily, where such equipment affords extensions to doctors' and surgeons' senses it is again aesthetic (the root of the word aesthetic is the ancient Greek *aesthesis* meaning "sense impression").

In this brief detour, I have already advertised the value of the medical humanities in the face of a dominant instrumental discourse and values complex – that of recognising the values complexes of ethics, aesthetics, politics, and the transcendental that take medical culture, its practitioners, pedagogies, and artefacts, beyond the instrumental or merely functional base to cultivate "meaning" beyond mere "information". Justice, form and beauty, and power issues are just as important to medicine and medical education as utility. Medical students are, to borrow Louis Althusser's term, "interpellated" into medical culture – its practices, semiotics, and languages – and then ideologically shaped, without protest or time to draw breath. Someone or something must then act within medicine and medical education as a critical presence advertising medicine as ideological, tempering its claims and excesses, and fundamentally questioning its practices where these seem to produce symptom – such as unacknowledged inflation leading to iatrogenesis, or medicine and surgery creating harm through unintentional error. As this book will spell out further, now we can see how important the medical humanities can be as reflexive and critical media within an often inflated, masculine, heroic, and instrumental medicine as the hubris of bioscience overshadows the need for intimacy, care, and empathy. In the classic criticism of objectification of patients, "Susan Smith" is reduced to "an invasive tumour" and "the lady in bed 3". In parallel, in the early days of adoption of the medical humanities, they were often considered as handmaidens to medicine and then also reduced, objectified, and slyly mocked or considered as irritant.

Back to a history of the future

The way that Michel Foucault proposes that we "do" history, as a tracing of the conditions of possibility for the emergence of any phenomenon, means that we can engage in a history of the future. By tracing the history of the medical humanities in a critically reflexive way we can stretch ourselves from the past and present into future scenarios with some confidence in quality of prediction. History becomes elastic and (for)giving rather than set in stone and foreboding.

Looping back to my potted history of the medical humanities, Penn State University developed a Department of Humanities within its medical school in the late 1960s, where students could choose to study medicine through the lenses of religion, history, philosophy, and literature. In 1969, *The Society for Health and Human Values* was established, merging in 1998 with the American Society for Bioethics and the Society for Bioethics Consultation to form the American Society for Bioethics and Humanities. So, formally, the disparate mess of the nascent medical humanities was brought under control by the bioethics movement. Bioethics and Law were tolerated by medics. The conditions of possibility for the emergence of a bioethics movement within medical education in North America were set by a practical incentive as noted earlier – increasingly, lawsuits were being brought against doctors and hospitals for malpractice. The basis of malpractice claims was often a question of perceived or actual ethical transgression.

This was the cover that would be used by innovative curriculum thinkers in medical schools, who would smuggle in a variety of medical humanities interests (as aesthetics and politics) under the acceptable (to hard-line biomedicine sceptics) umbrella of medical ethics, by now (the 1980s) accepted as necessary curriculum provision, often as "medical ethics + law". In the UK, the rebellious, yet adolescent, medical humanities would emerge from under the cover of the *British Medical Journal*'s special "Medical Ethics" issue to form an offshoot journal *Medical Humanities* and an organisation – The Association for Medical Humanities (AMH) – in 2000 (Evans and Greaves, 2001a, 2001b, 2002). While Adrian Hill's art therapy might be claimed as a UK-based "first" (are we suddenly in a race?), the UK's formal and more widespread adoption of the medical humanities lingered behind North America by about two decades. Having said that, medical humanities in medical education as curriculum content remained largely elective, and then taken up by few students. While medical humanities as a process element in curriculum (values permeating all curriculum provision, particularly anatomy and biomedical sciences) would be non-existent until the establishment of Peninsula Medical School in the UK in 2002 (see Chapter 3).

Typically, a discipline is established where it has an academic culture (a grant-supported research culture with a critical mass of publications), and an associated formal organisation running annual conferences and publishing a journal. [The UK Association for Medical Humanities was formalised in 2002 and held the first of its annual conferences in 2003. I joined the conference committee in 2004, was President 2013–16, and ran three annual conferences (2005, 2010 and 2015).] Legitimacy and due process often precedes academic quality or can act as a front for a potentially weak or splintered academic contribution.

The medical humanities gain a foothold through literary studies engaging medical education

Allow me to restate three of the conditions of possibility for the emergence of a medical humanities culture: first, the reaction against an increasingly scientific (and objectifying) biomedicine; second, the need for a voice to emerge from under the cover of a dominant bioethics culture that did not focus just on moral issues but on wider, general issues of quality of medical practice and related consequences of malpractice; and third, the existence of a small but influential core of medical humanities champions, mainly physicians passionate about medical education. Issues of quality then became a moral concern. Medical education and medical practice must be of a high standard. The baseline of acceptable practice – the mundane yet acceptable level of so-called "competence" – must be outstripped in aiming for capability, or what is often referred to as "excellence" (irritatingly, because the descriptor is so overused as to become meaningless, a "God-term" turned agnostic). Or a mundane "will-to-stability" is displaced by a desire for innovative "spearheads" of practice engaging a wider values system than the instrumental (Engeström 2018).

As we have seen, a voice of resistance against the mundane or purely instrumental in medicine first emerged in art therapies either side of the Atlantic. In Adrian Hill's work, he saw clinical care of recovering TB patients as adequate but lacking in quality. He didn't want his patients to simply while away the time – they were encouraged to create art, where technique was important. This visual-aesthetic intervention would develop its own culture as the profession of art therapy, but also, half a century later at the opening of the noughties would feed into the movement that would adopt the name of "health humanities" (Crawford, Brown and Charise 2020). Here, the entire project of bringing the arts and humanities to bear on issues of health and wellbeing would be democratised. The media of the arts and crafts would be treated not as the property of professional artists or scholars, but as the "available" arts, accessible to all.

Unfortunately, the baby of "technique" was thrown out with the bathwater of "participation". But, the entire spectrum of health and social care, including its participants – patients, professionals, and both paid and unpaid carers – were encouraged to participate in increasing the quality of healthcare and social wellbeing. Inclusivity was at the heart of this enterprise. Another spectre has haunted this movement, and it is echoed in the choice of the term "health" in health humanities. It is hard to criticise a movement that has wrapped itself in idealism, hope, and expectation. But the health humanities have, perhaps unconsciously, demonised "illness", such that "wellbeing" is the expectation that replaces Freud's 1895 observation (on mental health) that "much will be gained if we succeed in transforming your hysterical misery into common unhappiness" (Freud and Breuer 2004). Perhaps a better descriptor for the health humanities would be "healthcare humanities", shifting the focus from the idealism of wellbeing to the practice of healthcare itself. This can still be radically democratised, where unpaid carers give healthcare just as professional practitioners must. As I write this, with an eye to inclusion, the UK Association for Medical Humanities (AMH) has changed its name to the Association for Medical and Healthcare Humanities (AMHH).

In medical humanities, as opposed to the wider healthcare humanities spectrum, historically there would be a turn away from the visual arts, such as Hill's drawing and painting therapies, towards language and literature – primarily in the movement that came to be known as narrative-based medicine, as already noted. A group of North American literature scholars, including Anne Hudson Jones and Kathryn Montgomery Hunter, and later Tess Jones, Delese Wear, Lester Friedman, and Rita Charon (who was also a physician), would bring formal techniques from English Literature (such as "close reading") to bear on analysis of communication in healthcare contexts. A key focus would be on the patient's "story" that would complement the biomedical "chart" (Charon 2006). The patient's "story" would provide the embodied experience of symptom, rather than the literal and objective description of symptom as a platform for diagnosis and treatment (see Chapters 9 and 10). The shift would be away from the both quantitative data of the patient's chart (held as medicine's technical or informational capital) and the technical language of doctors and biomedical scientists, towards qualitative, language-based accounts of illness seen as the capital of patients.

The narrative-based medicine movement initiated by Charon in New York was preceded by a similar initiative in the UK (Greenhalgh and Hurwitz 1998, 1999; Launer 2002). Charon's movement came to overshadow that of the British medico-narrativists primarily because of the aggressive marketing of the Columbia University training programme, turning narrative medicine into a business enterprise (Bleakley and Neilson 2022). Economic values and virtues paralleled the aesthetic and ethical values and virtues promoted by narrative medicine as a response to bio-medicine's increasing instrumentalism. In essence, medical humanities became a business to be marketed, taking the edge off its critical potential. But we should not be surprised at this, given the context of the North American, Protestant-Capitalist tradition. Patients' illness stories have long provided capital for enterprise. We need only look at the explosion not only of doctors' autoethnographies and personal-confessional accounts, where patients' stories provide the meat of the content, but also of both TV medical soap operas (from Dr Kildare through ER and House MD) and "edutainment" documentaries.

Narrative-based medicine raises ethical considerations, where the reported patient "stories" run the risk of being the (re)constructions of the healthcare narrativists. This, rather than the capital of the patients themselves whose symptoms and utterances about those symptoms, often disjointed and exclamatory, are smoothed out into an orderly pattern of narrative with classic protagonists, plot, crisis, and denouement. Patients, perhaps, feel symptoms as much in space and place as in time; and perhaps lyric poetry (whose concern is more with space than time) is a better medium for appreciating and understanding the world of the patient than narrative. Yet spatial poetry and the poetic imagination have been wholly absorbed into the narrative medicine world, displaced, or overshadowed by temporal story (ibid.). Narrative medicine exponents will claim that the narrative is a co-construction of the patient's story and medical reading. But the fear is that the medical reading issues from a more powerful power base than the patient's account and so bends the patient's story to medicine's more technical needs.

To return to my running historical account, literature scholars – as early medical humanities proponents – pushed for medicine to simultaneously incorporate narrative knowing and awareness of social justice issues, led not by doctors with literature and social science as hobbies, but by literature and social science experts advising doctors. The first Institute of Medical Humanities was founded in 1973 at the University of Texas, Galveston, while the *Journal of Medical Humanities* was launched in 1979. In 1984, under the direction of the physician and ethicist Eric Cassell, a Hastings-commissioned report – "The Place of Humanities in Medicine" – was published. Another leader in the field, Edmund Pellegrino, marked 1984 (significant of course because of George Orwell's novel) as the year the medical humanities had come of age, ushering in a "post-evangelical" era, as Pellegrino described it. In other words, the medical humanities achieved the status of self-reflexivity rather than defensive justification and hard sell. Medical humanities had become "critical".

A decade later, in 1994, the New York School of Medicine established the first website dedicated to the medical humanities. Around the same time, Rita Charon established the first award-bearing *Program in Narrative Medicine* at Columbia University, New York, introduced above. To illustrate how sophisticated the interplay between narrative and medicine had become by the early 21st century, the reader is guided to the 2007 collection edited by Lee Gutkind, *Silence Kills: Speaking Out and Saving Lives*. This collection takes as its primary stimulus the emerging "patient safety" movement that aimed to challenge the culture of silence (and ignorance) that had developed around medical and surgical errors, to create a culture of transparency and learning. Its primary medium would become "creative nonfiction", illustrated particularly by the work of Abraham Verghese (1995, 1999, 2009, 2015), both physician and writer. Verghese was Director of the Centre for Medical Humanities and Ethics in San Antonio, Texas from 2002 to 2007.

At Columbia University (College of Physicians and Surgeons), New York, in 1991 the physician Arnold P. Gold and his psychologist wife Sandra Gold launched the Humanism in Medicine Award. The Gold Foundation has been central to the development of medical humanities in North America through its mission of supporting humanism across medicine, or authentic patient-centred practice. The Foundation does not embrace the more radical aspects of the arts, humanities and qualitative social sciences that might question habits and conventions in medicine, although it is deeply committed to a social justice agenda, challenging both inequities and inequalities. Paradoxically, while this social justice agenda is central to the work of the Gold Foundation, conservative "oath" rituals serving a common identification are pursued, such as the "White Coat Ceremony". This is anachronistic, where white coats have been dropped from most of medical practice. White coats (and, in part, stethoscopes) then maintain a symbolic purpose where their literal use has faded rapidly. White coats disappeared from medical practice some time ago in the UK, as did the wearing of ties, as both can harbour harmful bugs. Somewhere in amongst this cultural shift was the voice of Ignas Semmelweis, the

19th-century Hungarian physician who pioneered antiseptic procedures, but was at the time ridiculed for his experiments and conclusions that lack of basic procedures such as handwashing led to infection of patients.

The white coat is more a symbol of the acquired identity of the doctor through hard application and sacrifice – the acquisition of a spotless character too, a function of "professionalism" in medical education. Here, and again invoking a medical humanities approach, if we follow Michel Foucault's (1976) history of the "birth of the clinic" we can see how white coats became part of the symbolic armoury of doctors as a statement of sovereign power (and associated privilege) over patients. As the locus for medicine switched from home visits (where some power rested with the family) to the white space of the hospital and clinic, where power rested with medical professionals, so a set of symbolic objects would become associated with that power – specifically the white coat and stethoscope. Doctors (longer white coats) and medical students (shorter white coats) dressed this way as part of identity, separating them out from other healthcare workers such as nurses.

The introduction of the medical humanities into medicine and surgery curricula as a set of critical and therapeutic media would puncture such high-blown idealism to deal with the realities of a medicine and medical education, that, like all institutions would have fault-lines and contradictions as underlying illness, displayed in symptom. In the following chapter, I continue with a genealogy of the medical humanities, shifting geographically. While North America was instrumental in developing a critical mass for the establishment of the medical humanities, related activities were happening elsewhere in the world but on a smaller scale.

2

THE MEDICAL HUMANITIES COME OF AGE

More "origins" stories

To return to my potted history of the emergence of the medical humanities, the brief account given in the previous chapter of the rise of the medical humanities in North America conceals more than it reveals. First, it is given as a trouble-free historical narrative. But, of course, each historical event is fraught with difficulties, and events do not necessarily link to create a linear history. Again, we are in Foucauldian territory of a genealogical account tracking conditions of possibility for the emergence of a phenomenon. Accounts of scholars such as Kathryn Montgomery trying to establish literature programmes do not reveal the pain, hardship, and even humiliation that academic scholars often underwent at the hands of sceptical and sometimes bullying doctors, or a passive-aggressive medical culture with its associated unreconstructed management cultures. I have experienced this firsthand. Also, power struggles were rife inside institutions as issues such as gaining grants for research were played out. Medical school hierarchies often could not understand cultures of "soft" qualitative research, preferring "hard" evidence and numbers.

Some of this turmoil is captured in the key synoptic texts in the field. In what is called by its authors "the first textbook in medical humanities", Tom Cole, Nathan Carlin, and Ronald Carson (2015: 1) provide a simple rationale for the medical humanities – to provide a counterweight to the progressive "dehumanizing tendencies created by the unprecedented success of modern medicine and the commercialization of the healthcare system". Central to this is "biomedical reductionism". From this perceived dehumanisation, it is patients who are in distress. Cole and co-authors – notably an all-male team – provide 23 chapters justifying their claim, describing a compensatory curriculum for deep instrumentalising based on

DOI: 10.4324/9781003383260-3

interventions from history, literature and the arts, philosophy, and religion. Their approach may be seen as an example of the "dose effect" (Bishop 2008), where a dollop of the medical humanities supposedly compensates for a dehumanising biomedical science. But little thought is given to how we might rehabilitate the biomedical sciences. Patients, of course, are at the centre of this issue, but what if the institution and culture of medicine and its doctors are also in distress – suffering and symptomising? The premise of this otherwise ground-breaking text needed to be developed. The authors are also unapologetic for its blatant North American-centrism.

Cole and colleagues were also hasty in their primacy claim, for Tess Jones, Delese Wear, and Lester Friedman's *Health Humanities Reader* advertises a publication date of 2014. The text was bold enough to claim that "the health humanities (were) previously called the medical humanities". This collection, while again displaying North American-centrism, embraced a wide range of social justice issues grounded in health inequities and inequalities: disability studies, race, class and gender, access to treatment and care, and mental illness. It was altogether way more radical in its positioning than the Cole and colleagues' collection. The authors call for the health humanities – their preferred term of inclusivity – as a moral necessity, a responsible counterweight to biomedicine running away with its extraordinary potency, stripped of proper ethical concern and insensible when it comes to issues of social justice.

In 2016 a third weighty volume joined the two above: *The Edinburgh Companion to the Critical Medical Humanities*, edited by Anne Whitehead and Angela Woods, and showing a distinct UK-bias. This claims to have invented a "second wave" or "critical" medical humanities based on the notion of a complex "entanglement" of science, arts, and humanities. In this text, there is an explicit rejection any practical pedagogical interests for the medical humanities within medical education. Rather, there is a concern to grasp how medical cultures are historically and socially produced.

Advertising a challenge to North American-centric and UK-centric biases, my own edited volume, the *Routledge Handbook of the Medical Humanities* (Bleakley 2020a), also attempted to place pedagogical issues at the centre of the medical humanities with a rejection of "first wave" interests in medical humanities as compensatory for reductive biomedical science. Rather, the text works its way towards a "translational" position in which biomedical sciences, the arts, humanities, and qualitative social sciences can be seen to undermine their potentials where they adopt instrumentalism as the primary value. This transcends the tired "science vs arts" oppositional debate. Rather, as Kristeva and colleagues (2020) argue, the "medical humanities" might be taken as a bi-directional conversation between science and arts impinging on medicine that raises the qualities of each enterprise through translations, thus simultaneously addressing and embracing ethical, aesthetic, and political imperatives. This argument then focuses on axiological (values) issues rather than the usual epistemological (theory of knowledge) debates.

Returning to the historical theme of this section, in any case "origins" stories are always to be treated with scepticism, often offered rhetorically or with bias. For example, read any medical humanities text published in North America and you would think that the entire world was sandwiched between Los Angeles and New York (with the leftovers of the sandwich exported to Canada). Another origins story that challenges the imperialist one of the Northern Hemisphere are those of South America and Australia, a Southern Hemisphere account. In 1976, Anthony Moore, a surgeon working at the University of Melbourne, first used the term "medical humanities" in the published literature. Coincidentally, the University of La Plata medical school in Argentina established a medical humanities programme in the same year. I am sure that alternative histories of the origins of the medical humanities could be written from this Southern hemisphere perspective that would challenge the "origins" of the medical humanities claims based in North America and later in Canada.

The medical humanities in the UK, out of New Zealand

What has become known as a "first wave" medical humanities in the UK certainly originated in a strong medical ethics culture established during the 1960s and 1970s. The historical conditions of possibility for the rise of medical ethics are clear, as previously noted. Proliferation of technological and interventionist medicine throughout the 1960s and 1970s, including development of new drugs, new surgical techniques such as robotics, in vitro fertilisation, organ transplants and readily available contraception, raised a host of ethical issues. An unintended consequence of such rapid technological development was the decline in "hands-on" face-to-face medicine where areas such as diagnostic testing flourished, laboratory-based and imaging-based rather than bedside-based (as the physical examination, including auscultation, palpation, and percussion). This created a need to rekindle a more humane and caring medicine, inviting the development of the medical humanities as an ethical response to neglect of the patient as person. At the same time, the study of medical culture – as university-based academic medical humanities – would be stimulated as medical culture became entangled with ethics and of lay or public concern. The latter was stimulated by the rise of television, hospital-based soap operas (medi-soaps) such as "ER", "Casualty" and "Holby City" as well as medical and surgical documentaries. The study of medical culture itself, freed from entanglement with medical education, would form a "second wave" or "critical" medical humanities, flourishing particularly as the 20th century entered the 21st, as previously noted.

The development of the medical humanities world-wide is tied up with availability of grants to fund research and academic posts where salaries are funded by such grants. In the UK, this has been confounded by three main issues. First, funding for medical humanities has been restricted where the major funder, the Wellcome Trust, has chosen to support academic centres studying the culture of medicine, rather than the medical humanities in medical education (the second a far more pragmatic option). Funding for medical humanities in medical education is extremely sparse. Second, funding in medical schools for medical education has been shaped by a national exercise known as the Research Excellence Framework (REF) (previously the Research Assessment Exercise, or RAE). This places emphasis upon quantitative studies; and more, medical education is subsumed in wider categories of medical research or healthcare research, where its profile is squashed. All-in-all, medical humanities, set within medical education, has little or no profile within this set-up. And third, funding for medical humanities in university research settings is compromised by its inter-disciplinary nature. Funding tends to be dictated by conventional discipline boundaries, where inter-, trans-, or circum-disciplinary research (Bleakley 2014) is disadvantaged. As university departments return to the REF, this is organised by disciplines, so inter-disciplinary research is hard to situate. Thus, the growth of the medical humanities has been hampered not by the will of enthusiasts who wish to develop the area, but by organisational structures and strictures.

In the UK in 1993, the Wellcome Foundation organised a seminar on the arts in health, the first of its kind. Sir Kenneth Calman, a senior physician and arts and humanities enthusiast, was the Chief Medical Officer for England. Serendipitously, the General Medical Council (who offer guidance to medical schools on curricula) decided to overhaul the undergraduate medicine and surgery curriculum in the early 1990s (GMC 1993). *Tomorrow's Doctors* was published in a second incarnation in 2003, suggesting that beyond the core curriculum, optional modules could constitute up to a third of any English medical school's curriculum (GMC 2003). Such modules could (not should) include arts, humanities, and social sciences options. There were several drawbacks, however, to such a proposal. First, humanities were not explicitly encouraged as core, compulsory and assessed content. This would lead to medical humanities options being stereotyped as "light relief" from biomedical science and clinical skills studies, immediately devaluing the currency (as "edutainment"). Second, while medical schools were encouraged to develop humanities options, funding was not available for appointment of staff at senior levels (such as Professors) to develop such programmes, nor was there funding for research. For example, by 2002, only three dedicated full-time medical humanities posts existed across UK medical schools, all at junior level. The medical humanities initiative promised by an enthusiastic Calman was in a sense already dead in the water. It would be a struggle for medical schools to develop medical humanities programmes also where students were clamouring for sexy options such as "tropical medicine", "sports medicine" and "expedition medicine".

Despite these blocks, momentum did grow. By 2005, Peninsula Medical School (UK) had appointed Visiting Professors in Fine Art, Music and History, and an Associate Professor in Ethics and Philosophy of Medicine, plus a full-time lecturer in Medical Humanities, and several research staff. As Professor in Medical Education, by 2007 I had also taken on the role of lead in medical humanities that was established as core, compulsory and assessed provision. Within an overall medical education remit, I was able to acquire funding (particularly from the European Union) for research projects that embraced ethics and medical humanities elements. For example, a multi-disciplinary project aiming to improve team process in operating theatres embraced both film and performance studies, where we were able to link with the nearby Falmouth University's art school resources to develop collaborative projects. Actor patients worked with operating theatre nurses, surgeons, and anaesthetists to act out prepared scripts as typical scenarios advertising patient safety incidents. These were professionally filmed in a television studio and used for teaching purposes. Meanwhile, operating theatre teams were videotaped live at work and professionally edited selections shown as a basis for debriefing of a day's list. Issues of "identity" and "performance" ranked high amongst practitioners' interests (this was, after all, "theatre"), as did issues of democratic working habits underpinning patient safety (Allard et al. 2007, 2011; Bleakley 2006, 2013; Bleakley et al. 2004, 2013). Thus, aesthetic, ethical, and political issues were immediately raised beyond functional values and concerns.

Returning to the establishment of the medical humanities in UK medical education, Robin Philipp, a public health consultant, had organised the first medical humanities conference outside North America, in Wellington, New Zealand in 1994. Two years later, the first New Zealand narrative in medicine conference was held in Auckland. Philipp was later to move to the UK, bringing his medical humanities expertise with him. During his time as CMO of England (1991–98), Kenneth Calman pursued an agenda for medical education to embrace the arts and humanities, but his philosophy was idealistic, as noted above. He saw the value of the arts as creating a kind of warm glow around medicine as the public pursued "wellbeing" and "happiness". This was a long way from the vision of many artists, following Nietzsche's philosophy for example, that the arts should be troublesome, irksome – agitating, upsetting and revolutionary – more likely to cause discomfort, even illness and distress, as they pursued the aim of questioning normativity, habit, or the status quo where this led to mundane situations. As Aristotle said, the unexamined life was not worth living.

This gadfly role for the medical humanities was not welcome across medical schools. Medical educators, especially clinicians, mostly did not want an irritant questioning the values and practices of medicine. Medicine, a stressful occupation, looked to the arts and humanities for a means of relaxation, diversion, a switching off from the hard stuff of science. But core medical humanities devotees saw value in the medical humanities as a standing aspect of the core curriculum that would provide a running critique of medical education's ideological interpellation – the unacknowledged repetition of instrumental values within medicine, at the expense of other values perspectives. Rather, the medicine curriculum authors sought "rounded" doctors – wholesome fellows exercising empathy and person-centred care. Nothing wrong with this – such humanitarian values had been modelled by the Gold Foundation in the USA for many years, as noted in the previous chapter.

But this is too cosy for most artists and critical thinkers who want a blistering aesthetics and wide-eyed social justice, characteristic, for example, of the best of performance art.

Philipps and Calman co-organised the first Windsor Conference in 1998 where arts in medicine would no longer be marginalised, but would adopt, for example, therapeutic and supportive roles. In the second Windsor conference in 1999, one of the organisers, Robin Downie, would say that "art can be counterproductive if it is done for the wrong reasons. The typical artist is, for example, not a good health role model!" Apart from the stereotyping, this reveals a timidity inherent to medical humanities that would characterise much of its early history in the UK. The arts were characterised as a "healing force" rather than as a force problematising the very notion of "healing" itself (returning us to Nietzsche's view that illness can be a productive state). At the 1999 second Windsor conference, where key medical humanities movers and shakers from North America were invited, it was admitted by the conference organisers that UK medical humanities were "20 years behind North America", as noted in the previous chapter.

This was all to change within the next decade as the UK Association for Medical Humanities was developed, with its associated annual conference and British Medical Journal (BMJ) affiliated journal *Medical Humanities,* coupled with the curriculum initiatives modelled by Swansea University, University College London and Peninsula Medical School and later medical schools such as Bristol, Durham, Warwick, Southampton, Brighton (Sussex), Leicester, Nottingham, Manchester, Glasgow, Aberdeen, Keele, Leeds, Imperial College, and Sheffield. But prior to these initiatives, in 1997 Martyn Evans, a philosopher, and David Greaves, a doctor with a PhD in ethics, set up a MA in medical humanities at Swansea University in Wales (Evans and Greaves 2001b). Evans would go on to edit the BMJ *Medical Humanities* journal, launched in 2000; and in 2002 the Association for Medical Humanities (AMH) was formed, with Evans and President, and two doctors – Jane Macnaughton and Brian Hurwitz – and Anne Borsay, a medical historian, as its co-founders.

In 1998 two London-based General Practitioners, Deborah Kirklin and Richard Meakin, established a Centre for Medical Humanities at the Royal Free Hospital and University College, London. This provided a high-water mark for medical humanities thinking and practice at the time, with a focus upon literature and film. The unit developed a one-year intercalated BSc in medical humanities for medical students and several postgraduate programmes. A decade later, the University would close the programme in a management-led rationalisation of resources, now often referred to as "efficiency". Peninsula (Universities of Exeter and Plymouth), Durham (Wellcome-funded Centre for Medical Humanities) and King's College London (Centre for Literature and Medicine) would pick up the baton. As detailed in the following chapter, Peninsula modelled integration of medical humanities into an undergraduate medicine programme; Durham developed a thriving research centre with several projects looking at the study of medical culture and medical phenomena, but not specifically medical education; and King's developing a Master's programme in Literature and Medicine, and a doctoral supervision programme. In parallel, a History of Medicine Centre had long been established at Exeter University and this received significant funding from the Wellcome Trust to study medical culture, expanding into a broader medical humanities centre in time. Ironically, while Exeter hosted a medical humanities programme at the medical school, a separate Centre for Bioethics, and the History of Medicine Centre, despite many efforts, the three enterprises would never link to form a superpower.

The medical humanities, in one form or another, are now common across medical schools globally. I will refrain from listing institutions that provide some model or other of the medical humanities – these stretch across Europe, Asia, and the Pacific Rim. For example, at the Sorbonne in Paris, a Master's degree in bio-medical humanities has been established where medical students can study humanities, while humanities students can study medicine. The programme is based on George Canguilhem's (1989) contention that medicine is an art flourishing at the crossroads of several sciences (physiology, biochemistry, and anatomy). A new medical humanities organisation – the *Institut La Personne en médicine* – has recently been established in the Paris City University spawning a research culture, conferences, and website (https://u-paris.fr/la-personne-en-medecine/institut/). Italy has long had a thriving medical humanities culture based on the notion that medical students and doctors should have a rounded education incorporating the arts and humanities. Both India and Sri Lanka are also developing medical humanities programmes. In parallel, there are now at least half a dozen established medical humanities journals worldwide.

The global medical humanities

The "Global Medical/Health Humanities" has become an unfortunate and rather meaningless descriptor, devoid of any critical content such as focusing upon North American imperialism in the field. A better tack might be to focus upon inclusivity in medical humanities, where issues such as gender bias, stereotyping and exclusion of minorities are addressed. A 2022 edition of the BMJ journal *Medical Humanities* focused on the global medical humanities, addressing topics such as the legacies of colonialism shown in racism, and other contributing factors to health disparities such as gender bias, ableism, and language elitism. Importantly, methods of inquiry are now more commonly seen as shaped by cultural inflections. This challenges the longstanding bias in research methods established by Northern hemisphere imperialism, spearheaded by North American interests. This legacy also privileges the quantitative over the qualitative.

The medical humanities should be considered as a liberatory global text, challenging a colonising or neo-imperialism "expressive of Western culture" (Hooker and Noonan 2011). An illustrative example is the attempt to foster eye contact in small group work with native Japanese students in a culture where direct eye contact is considered rude (Bleakley, Bligh and Browne 2011). Similarly, from a medical humanities perspective, Western/ Northern European models of "empathy" may be (mis)applied in, say, an African or Indian subcontinent context of medical education where the "sensitivity" in Northern European "empathy" is by-passed in more direct encounters, possibly even considered bullying or rude in terms of, say, a North American, Canadian, or northern European model of empathic encounter (Eichbaum et al. 2022). In a black South African context, northern hemisphere views of individualism and competitiveness are considered strange, where Ubuntu (supportive collectivism) is the primary mode of relating. Further, how will an Islamic-based medical humanities deal with such Western cultural bias (Abdel-Halim and AlKattan 2012)? In a marked shift from the positivist philosophy that influenced medical education for more than a century, world medical educators now realise the significance of spiritual values beyond the instrumental that dominates science and the humanistic that pervades models of patient care and clinical-communication skills. This is particularly acute when it comes to issues of end-of-life care and terminal illness. Western medical educators can learn from the medicine taught and practiced during the Islamic civilisation era as a vivid example of the unity of the two components of medical knowledge: natural sciences and spiritually inflected humanities.

In terms of course developments, for example, St Bartholomew's (Barts) and the London School of Medicine and Dentistry run a one-year intercalated BSc in Global Medical Humanities that will,

> give you a global perspective on key debates in medicine and healthcare (e.g., COVID-19, transplants, disasters, mental health, disability) across a range of cultural contexts. Our Medical Humanities programme explores global literary and cultural objects (including fiction and non-fiction, film, visual art) and urges us to rethink our understanding of care, health, risk and vulnerability. You will be challenged to reflect on the complex relationship between medicine and healthcare and social inequalities, human rights, environmental and humanitarian crises, and questions of ethics.

The promise is that through topics such as "Madness Past and Present, Film and Disability, World Literature and Ethics, and Language and Communication", students will develop a "self-reflexive medical practice". These are terms out of contemporary arts and humanities and not fully developed within medicine or medical education. But these are the topics that should be compulsory within a medicine undergraduate curriculum. The media used to discuss these topics (film, literature, language) can readily be incorporated into a biomedicine curriculum: such as a film about Henrietta Lacks or the Tuskegee Study of Untreated Syphilis; Abraham Verghese's (1995) account of the early days of the AIDS epidemic in rural America (*My Own Country*); or a study of the uses of metaphor in medicine (Bleakley 2017).

In North America, the Massachusetts Institute of Technology (MIT) "Global Health and Medical Humanities" initiative is currently led by an anthropologist, Erica Caple James, and promises inter-disciplinary study of medicine and healthcare through political, economic, social, and cultural lenses. In her doctoral dissertation James (2010) herself took a critical look at the work of aid agencies in Haiti in 1994, following the political coup. She found that while some aid programmes did help Haitians on the ground, others merely reinforced existing social divisions (https://betterworld.mit.edu/global-health-and-medical-humanities/). There is a moral here for the development of medical humanities programmes within medical schools. Too often such programmes are formed on terms set by the dominant biomedical discourse and its institutional representations. As noted earlier, this sets up an expectation that the medical humanities will refrain from acting as an internal critique of restrictive biomedicine, or of medical education based on reductive instrumentalism and grounded in learning through simulation (such as clinical and communication skills). In Chapter 4, I outline how the medical humanities can act not only as a critical friend to reductive biomedicine and clinical/communication skills training, but also as a therapist in addressing longstanding symptoms within medical culture clustered around reductionism. In most medical schools, such an approach would be defused at root.

The medical humanities were always in danger of falling foul of hierarchy embodied in the exercise of superiority of medicine over other healthcare professions, and further embedded in the perceived superiority of North America over other continents. Where the Brits suggested that they lagged 20 years behind North America, both failed to see key early developments in the medical humanities in other parts of the world such as Argentina and New Zealand.

Now there is a truly global and collaborative medical/ health humanities culture. For example, the relatively recently formed Canadian Association for Health Humanities (CAHH), with its annual conferences and academic networks, was founded on the model of the UK Association for Medical Humanities. Indeed, Canada can now, arguably, be seen as the epicentre of medical/health humanities developments working in parallel with medical education. The past four winners of the bi-annual Karolinska Prize for Medical Education (medical education's Nobel equivalent) are based in Canada, originally having worked in the Wilson Centre affiliated with the University of Toronto and now having moved on to other posts: Brian Hodges, Lorelei Lingard, Glenn Regehr, and Kevin Eva.

The UK's health humanities network meanwhile has developed independently from the established medical humanities network, and now holds its own conferences, initiates research and has a website that advertises its qualities in terms of independence from the yoke of the "medical" (https://www.nottingham.ac.uk/research/groups/mental-health/old-site-content/projects/health-humanities.aspx). Interestingly, the health humanities movement has also poached wholesale from the medical humanities movement and dressed it in new clothes – see for example: https://healthhumanitiesconsortium.com/about/, where a "timeline" for the development of the health humanities is in fact a timeline developed by Tess Jones (from Denver, Colorado) and myself to describe a history of the medical humanities.

The translational medical humanities

Broadly, the modern art therapy seed attributed to Adrian Hill and Margaret Naumberg had a direct line of development into professional art therapy, requiring postgraduate qualification. Such therapies are used widely in hospital and recovery/ community settings, particularly in mental health. By the beginning of this century a movement, seeded by Paul Crawford in the UK (a literature graduate who had worked in mental health and become an influential academic) rejected the professional insularism of arts therapies. Crawford called for a public, de-professionalised, democratic arts therapies movement in which the art medium was secondary to the therapy. Participants needed no expertise in the medium. This also moved the use of arts and humanities away from its historical base in medicine to all healthcare practices (including the de-professionalised practice of "family carer"). Here, the "health humanities" were born (Crawford et al. 2010, 2015; Crawford, Brown and Charise 2020) as a democratic or inclusive gesture. There was, however, some evident confusion. The medical humanities movement in the UK had never claimed to be exclusive and many participants in events and conferences were from healthcare professions other than medicine. The term "medical" was not used in a divisive or autocratic way. "Health" humanities have similar naming problems. As noted, a better, but more cumbersome term would be "healthcare" humanities, for the "health" humanities surely deal with illness or sickness as not only an ever-present aspect of the human condition, but one that many recognise as ground for creativity.

Noted previously, as the medical/ health humanities developed, so two major initiatives emerged within the UK and Europe. In the UK, a "critical" medical humanities developed that was reflexive and inquiring. University-based researchers and academics working within the field of the study of medical cultures (the history and anthropology of medicine, bioethics, medicine and literature, medicine, and performance studies, and so forth) were not particularly interested in application of their studies to medical education. A split then arose between medical humanities in medical education and the medical humanities as the academic, inter-disciplinary study of medical cultures. Both camps have made claims upon the descriptor "critical" medical humanities (Bates, Bleakley and Goodman 2014, Whitehead and Woods 2016).

The "critical" aspect is grounded in the legacy of Immanuel Kant's (Schmidt 1996: 58–64) plea for individuals to free themselves from the dogmas imposed by the Church and State, to cultivate independent thinking. Such thinking is both rational and critical. Every idea is scrutinised, and values are reflexively tested – "what is it that I value, and why do I value it? Why do I think this way, what shapes me? What are the alternatives to my way, and have I thought these through?" Such self-interrogation breaches tradition, orthodoxy, and ideology. This is further grounded in the 19th-century German Romantic movement with its inquiry into "what is self?", reinforced by Hegel's idealist philosophy of the inevitable evolution of the human mind (through dialectical thinking: movements of thesis, antithesis, and synthesis) from darkness to illumination realised as Spirit or identification with a commonly held ideal (Wulf 2022). This of course has become the meaning of democracy. First, the mind is shorn from ideological dictation by others such as Church dogma; then it becomes self-reflexive and self-illuminating in meta-cognition; and finally, it joins a collective mind of reflexive inspiration that is identification with Hegelian Spirit as a tolerant intersubjectivity, or common understanding of human freedom.

A similar reflexivity arc has shaped the "critical" medical humanities, whose primary role is to interrogate medicine's values and assumptions, drawing on methods such as various forms of historical, anthropological, or philosophical approaches. There is a double interrogation and reflexivity at work: first, that of addressing medicine's habits and traditions to frame new ways of thinking about, and with, medicine and medical education; and second, to address the values shaping and informing one's own method of inquiry. In a review of medical humanities provision in Canadian medical schools, Kidd and Connor (2008) define the medical humanities as "reflection and critical thinking about the human body and mind". Medicine alone does not do this. Allan Peterkin and colleagues (2020) have updated Kidd and Connor's original review, where 12 of the 17 medical schools in Canada now report some form of medical/ health humanities activity within their curricula. But the core impulse is Hegelian – dialectical inquiry and ongoing critique and re-building of foundations, affording a paradoxical architectural imagination at work within medical humanities that refuses "foundations" at the same time as it respects processional history.

What the critical medical humanities have achieved is the better understanding of specific phenomena such as language use in medical contexts, but they have perhaps failed to capture how clinical practice itself, the heart of medicine, can be transformed. Medical practices remain stubbornly hierarchical, masculine-heroic and individualist despite advertising patient-centredness and inter-professional teamwork as key.

Where the critical medical humanities have excelled at analysis, it can be said that they have failed to translate across to the experiential worlds of healthcare practitioners and their patients. Where Freud's psychoanalytic insights would be hollow without psychoanalytic method, Derrida's insights into the limits of language and the importance of "horizons" would be sterile without Julia Kristeva's practical examples of preverbal "speech" (semiotics) engaging the abject, the absent and the inexplicable in both chronic and acute social contexts such as the suffering of migrants as they attempt to adapt to unfamiliar cultures. This adaptation is cast as a form of translation. It is not only linguistic and cultural translation, but also a translation of psyche at an unconscious level, as explored below. Moving on from a "critical" medical humanities, Kristeva and colleagues (2020) have developed the "translational" medical humanities as a "third wave".

Kristeva's work might be seen as the seed for the development of medical humanities in French medicine and medical education – initially resisted as a distinct approach because French medicine has always regarded itself as intimately bound with a humanities tradition [similarly with Italian medicine (Fieschi et al. 2013)]. Noted above, the Medical Humanities Institute of The Person in Medicine Institute of the City University of Paris was inaugurated in 2020 and celebrated with the publication of a text: *Les Humanités médicale. L'engagement des sciences humaines et sociales en medicine* (Lefève, Thoreau and Zimmer 2020). This may be regarded as the flagship organisation for the medical humanities in France, running regular seminars and conferences.

To return to Julia Kristeva, she has been working with psychiatrists and social workers in helping young, displaced persons (refugeed due to war or political conflict) to settle in Paris. Their work is necessarily "translational" in the sense that they are literally translating across languages to help the displaced person to adapt. But more, they are working with translations across cultures and translations between unconscious and conscious process in unfamiliar settings (Kristeva et al 2020). To bring the tender developmental and unconscious architecture of young persons into unfamiliar cultural territory demands nourishing and careful support, for ruptures are inevitable. Further, there is translation to be pursued between the preverbal, regressive states – that young people find themselves trapped in when socially harassed, at the receiving end of prejudice, or plain misunderstood – and the verbal, communicative states of the fully functioning adult.

Kristeva (1982) herself, a Bulgarian by birth, has seen translation across cultures as key to her work as a psychoanalyst. This is particularly evident in her interest in the influence of early mother-child relationships focused on the pre-verbal in children, where articulation is affect-laden and non-verbal. Here, moving on from the work of Donald Winnicott and others on the child's early relation to transitional objects (such as teddy bears and other toys), Kristeva (ibid.) focuses on the child's relationship with the abject, or horror. It is in unresolved issues with the abject – whatever is cast off as disgusting or unbearable – that the major developmental issues rest. In translating this personal developmental dynamic to a cultural stage, Kristeva and colleagues inquire into how the repression of horror, the abject, affects young refugees. For they have seen wars and violence, torture, rapes and murders, and the underbellies of refugee camps. Their transitional objects may have been guns or knives. More, this has been impressed upon a tender, developing psyche where much has been repressed, so that such immigrants often displace disturbing and unresolved unconscious impulses into errant, often anti-social, behaviours. In migration, such young people are fundamentally rendered insensible, or blunted.

This topic is central to medical education and yet ignored in practice. Particularly in *Educating Doctors' Senses through the Medical Humanities* (Bleakley

2020b) I argue that initial medical education offers a paradoxical education into insensibility. This is a "compulsory mis-education", to draw on the title of Paul Goodman's (1966) classic on the unintended consequences of schooling. Traditionally, in undergraduate medical education, while sensibility and sensitivity are desired for physical examination, patient contact and diagnosis, sensibility (literally an education of the senses in learning close noticing) is eroded. First, through the initiation ritual of learning anatomy through dissection, and second in learning clinical and communication skills in the bubble of simulation rather than in live work-based clinical learning. The rationale is that medical students must dull themselves to the abject – the horrors of death, illness, and bodily and mental wounding, gaining emotional distance from patients. This dis-identification or emotional insulation keeps one from tipping into emotional distress through over-identification and associated stress. However, I show how these are crude strategies.

Learning how to "dull" or "anaesthetise" oneself elegantly has been well documented in psychoanalytic technique since Freud. This depends upon mastering the psychological effects of counter-transference and counter-resistance. The whole basis of forming a therapeutic relationship with a patient in medicine, or a client in psychotherapy, or one of Kristeva's (and colleagues') distressed and displaced young persons is to manage their transference and resistance dynamics while seeing through your own. This is far more sophisticated than the crude techniques used in medical education to produce "emotional insulation" in medical students that rely on exposure techniques promising "resilience" without learning any psychological acumen. The level of empathy loss, cynicism, burnout, anxiety, depression and suicidal ideation amongst later years medical students and junior doctors shows clearly that such blunt medical education techniques have not worked. Medical students need to learn psychological acumen, or Kristeva and colleagues' medical humanities as "translational" practices. Where "absorption" into a new culture (Islamic youth into a mix of French Catholicism and humanistic republicanism for example) is another example of ideological interpellation, naturally such youth will resist, engaging in acting out and other defensive behaviours. Medical education (through the medical humanities) can learn much from this scenario as it teaches strategies of doctor-patient interactions. To call these interactions "communication skills" is insulting, for such transactions move beyond skills and competences to looser and more indeterminate capabilities (always in the process of development) that centre on semiotics, or meaning in, and through, language embracing signs and symbols. Such language at core is emotional and expressive, or cathartic (Heron 1977, 2001).

Again, a transactional and translational relationship to the abject (death, illness, disease, cruelty, despair) is central to learning how to be a doctor and the primary techniques to be learned are grounded in psychoanalytic psychotherapy post-Freud. In medical education, as the abject is mishandled, so it is repressed and returns in a distorted form as symptom. Medicine itself suffers from a masculinist, heroic, impulsive individualism that can lead to medical error as it resists collaborative teamwork widely shown to improve patient safety. This restrictive practice – rather than reflective practice – produces symptoms of empathy loss, cynicism, and dis-identification (Bleakley 1999). Medical students remain, in Freudian terms, in an arrested state of development, stuck in the anal stage ("hanging on"/retention or "letting go"/expulsion at the child's will rather than in recognition of the adult social convention) – the acceptable "frontstage" of a condition that has the abject as its backstage or place of horrors – where characteristic behaviours are controlling and lack reflexivity. Language forms here are grounded in the indicative (telling) rather than the subjunctive mood (discussing). Individualism and hierarchy trump collectivism (working in democratic teams). A prime psychological characteristic is intolerance of ambiguity or uncertainty.

These symptoms can, however, be treated. Transitions can be made from anality to adult genitality or genuine sharing, collaboration, and democratic practices. In Kristeva's terms, the preverbal semiotic and the abject that accompanies this do not constitute a regressive trap (medical culture at its worse), but a springboard for insight (such conditions forming the very field that is needed to work empathically across differing transactions with suffering always as the horizon).

One characteristic of regressive anality is hanging on to one's prejudices. Thus, Kristeva and colleagues articulate "translational" medical humanities as a complex in which boundary crossings between the biomedical sciences and the arts/ humanities/ qualitative social sciences are essential. This is a grown-up view. One ventures into territories of the "other" to understand their world views. Eventually, one incorporates such views into one's own world in learning adaptation, rather than persistently assimilating the "other" into one's fixed position (again, a characteristic of the anal, regressed outlook). For our shell-shocked, and culturally confused young immigrant such smooth transition from anality to grown-up (democratic) genitality may be a leap too far. Acting out, as the child does, is likely to be the primary response. This is prior to therapeutic intervention, where transitions to adult play are required, as contracts of settlement in an unfamiliar culture. But integration does not demand subservience. Rather, it can invite participation through bringing one's talents and personality to bear on that host culture. There are distinct parallels here with the marriage of biomedical science and the medical humanities.

Fourth wave medical humanities

If Kristeva and colleagues have articulated a "third wave" medical humanities focused on issues of translation across bioscience and the arts and humanities, I suggest a "fourth wave" medical humanities that is a psychoanalytic strategy addressing medicine's symptoms. It is an extension of the "third wave" view and is fully developed in Chapters 5 and 6. This, in turn, advertises a return of the repressed. Again, at its core, through medical education or medical pedagogic strategies, medicine represses – or blunts – the necessary and everyday abject met as symptom in patients and populations that would otherwise be overwhelming for medical students. This is seen in developing masculine-tinged heroism, cynicism, and suspension of empathy as emotional insulation. These keep the dragons of the abject at bay. A primary theatre for the playing out of such tactics is learning anatomy through cadaver dissection. Here, historically, medical students have found ways to repress emotional flux by objectifying the cadaver, developing camaraderie around deflecting disgust, and developing (often unsavoury) humour (Bleakley 2020b).

Such blunting of sensibility and sensitivity – characteristically registered and investigated as empathy decline and rise in cynicism – creates a culture shaped by the return of the repressed that cries out for analytic intervention to recover the sensitive body of biomedicine that rests beneath the carapace of cultural ego defence mechanisms.

Traditional masculine, heroic and rational (anti-affective) medicine is bolstered through stiff hierarchies operating across healthcare. Medicine needs to be both democratised and feminised, and then brought into the realms of "critical" health studies where it gains self-insight or psychotherapeutic acumen. While the high rates of burnout, disaffection, cynicism, depression, anxiety, and suicidal ideation seen in medicine can be partly explained by structural factors (such as resource starvation; and an inability to manage an open, complex, non-linear, adaptive system at the edge of chaos through linear, closed, engineering principles), they are better explained as poor psychotherapeutic acumen amongst doctors. This, in turn, is a legacy of an ineffective or blunted medical education.

And here, I have casually dropped in a major factor that the medical humanities can educate for: medicine as an open, complex, adaptive system at the edge of chaos – and ready to transition spontaneously to a higher order of complexity – that must be framed as such for its management. However, medicine and medical education alike regress to treating their worlds as closed, linear systems that can be engineered. Hence the constant reduction to instrumentalism (again, fixed "competences" and technical "skills" rather than fluid "capabilities") that I see as a symptom of medical education's restricted horizon, rather than a pedagogical advance, as often claimed. I will have much more to say about a systems approach as one of medical humanities' major contributions to medical education in Chapter 6.

At this point I will remind the reader that it is worth recalling that Charles Darwin never drew on machine or engineering metaphors to discuss evolution. Rather, evolving bodies are complex, ambiguous, and malleable. As medicine has progressed, so machine (body as advanced plumbing and wiring, etc.) and martial (medicine as war) metaphors have dominated (Bleakley 2015). Patients remain as complex, adaptive systems trapped in an entropic world (we are all ailing and moving towards death). We can be engineered instrumentally to a degree (look at interventional cardiology, or many pharmaceutical interventions), but medicine has its limits. It is at these limits that the medical humanities show their power, grappling with existential issues such as why do people deliberately seek to harm their bodies and psyches (bad lifestyles, bad diet, pursuing dangerous and life threatening "leisure" activities, piling on anxiety through overwork) at the same time as they seek medical interventions to heal their bodies and psyches? In parallel, why do we tolerate the structural production of poverty, illness, and disease as a product of inequity, inequality, and social injustice, when many of these injustices could be addressed through the redistribution of capital and resources? Medical education is largely failing to address these issues, many of them now wrapped in the health implications of the climate crisis (Bleakley 2021). But, as this book describes, the medical humanities are addressing such issues.

3

CORE, COMPULSORY, AND ASSESSED

Medical humanities innovations at Peninsula
Medical School

The medical humanities gain traction

In October 2003, the prestigious American journal *Academic Medicine* – dedicated
to the rapidly expanding field of medical education research – devoted an issue
solely to the medical humanities in medical education. It did not offer a critical
approach, but rather catalogued developments of medical humanities initiatives
in medical schools internationally. The bulk of entries were from North America,
reflecting an on-the-ground reality that North American medical humanities programmes were more populous than other global movements, but also signalled a
nationalistic bias (and in some ways a colonising of the medical humanities culture,
as discussed in the previous chapter). At this time, the medical humanities were
lauded by many proponents as "coming of age". The reality was different – the
medical humanities remained handmaiden to medicine and offered little in the way
of pedagogical innovation within medical education. Mainly, the undergraduate
curriculum allowed medical humanities in through the back door, as electives studied by relatively small numbers of students.

Medical schools were making little concerted effort to develop the medical
humanities as core, integrated, and assessed curriculum content – the grown-up
view. Indeed, biomedically science-oriented critics of medical humanities had their
foes over a barrel, demanding of them to provide hard evidence, or proof, of the
educational impact of medical humanities initiatives. And more, of the even harder
to prove knock-on effect of improvement of patient care and safety. Further, for
credibility, proof must be quantitative, evidence open to statistical analysis. This
forced research down the avenue of numbers-based inventories and scales, rather
than experiential accounts gleaned from qualitative analysis of videotaped practice, and other innovative ethnographies. Thus, medical humanities proponents

DOI: 10.4324/9781003383260-4

were forced into a corner, bullied by the very instrumental, quantitative-driven, and reductive approach of biomedical science that the medical humanities fundamentally challenged. Many medical humanities proponents in medical schools were afraid of losing their jobs, such as qualitative social scientists uneasy with the quantitative "hard evidence" approach, employed to help with areas such as teaching communication skills and professionalism. How does an English literature academic get her head around levels of statistical significance as opposed to narrative testimony for example?

Against this background, *Academic Medicine* organised a conference in New York to launch the special issue and to provide an opportunity for an international audience to share their experiences in the field. Almost all delegates were from medical schools developing medical humanities programmes. As expected, almost all were North American and despite the celebratory atmosphere (after all we were temporarily out of the grip of the biomedical sceptics, enjoying the company of like-minded people) almost all were fundamentally dispirited about the progress the medical humanities were making in medical schools. This was reflected, for example, in a scandalous lack of senior academic appointments (at Professorial level) in the medical humanities globally. Further, there was difficulty in gaining traction to move from elective to compulsory study.

I was there with colleagues to represent the newly established UK Peninsula Medical School. We had our first intake of medical students in 2002 and had planned an ambitious medical humanities programme, unique (we think) to any medical school at the time. We planned to make the medical humanities – and we would spend plenty of time debating what that term meant – core, compulsory and assessed syllabus *content* in the curriculum (Bleakley et al. 2006). But more, we would frame the medical humanities as a formative *process* within the curriculum. We were fortunate to be planning the new curriculum as several helpful external forces converged. For the first time, the England General Medical Council (GMC) introduced a directive that medical undergraduate programmes should include medical humanities components; senior staff in our new school were supportive of the medical humanities initiative; and as the medical school initially had a small faculty, through careful recruitment, thoughtful staff development and meticulous curriculum planning we were able to create an educational climate supportive of a positive conversation between anatomy, biomedical sciences, clinical and communication skills, and the arts and humanities. Serendipity indeed!

Viewing curriculum as process (for example of identity formation) as well as content (formal syllabus), we developed ways in which the curriculum could be experienced by students and faculty as a parallel series of texts: primarily aesthetic, ethical and political, but also, for example, historical. Our pedagogical guide was the curriculum reconceptualisation movement, based on the pioneering work of William Pinar (for example 2004, 2019). For readers unfamiliar with this approach, here is an all-too-brief introduction. It serves to remind us that the medical humanities in medical education primarily pose *pedagogical* questions.

We were also careful to reflexively question our intentions in introducing a medical humanities programme to the undergraduate medicine and surgery curriculum by asking, in an early paper, what are the dangers of the medical humanities becoming an imperative ("you will be humane!") rather than an invitation (Petersen et al. 2008). We wanted to move beyond evangelism, and to create a different kind of contract in particular with anatomy and biomedical science faculty that would benefit both parties.

Curriculum reconceptualisation

Let us then take a short diversion to explain and briefly explore curriculum reconceptualisation. It was central to our curriculum planning at Peninsula, that took the medical humanities to the heart of the undergraduate medicine and surgery curriculum. Where I describe the medical humanities as core, compulsory and assessed, this is a long way from most medical humanities curriculum interventions. These again tend to be electives or non-assessed modules, an aspect of syllabus or curriculum *content*. A curriculum *process* approach, in contrast, sees all curriculum content (syllabus) as subject to ways of learning and experiencing that produce identities. "Thinking with" the medical humanities spectrum fundamentally offers ways of intensifying the quality of a largely biomedical science and clinical and communication skills curriculum by adding other values positions to its baseline value position of instrumentalism or functionalism. This is easy to understand through an analogy: the poet T.S. Eliot (1934) describes the transition from mere "information" to "knowledge" and then "wisdom" as the essence of poetry: "Where is the wisdom we have lost in knowledge? Where is the knowledge we have lost in information?"

In this pedagogical approach, the medical humanities afford media through which curriculum content can be lived or experienced (as curriculum process) as it is reflected upon, critiqued, and continually revised. Curriculum reconceptualisation then turns the noun "curriculum" (a "thing" that, again, is in effect a syllabus) into the verb *currere*, meaning to "run the course of study" (a process of learning and gaining of identity). More, this process is characterised as an open, adaptive, non-linear, complex system at the edge of chaos (and subject to spontaneous reformulation at a higher level of complexity), rather than a closed, linear system open to instrumental engineering. The content approach to curriculum has also produced the pedagogical contradiction that learning becomes driven by assessment, where students focus not on knowledge and wisdom, but on information.

Paradoxically, while the medical humanities *in* medical education have developed or stalled in their various ways, the medical humanities *as* medical education have never gained a foothold. This stems in part from the rather strange, and embarrassing, position that medical educators, clinicians, biomedical scientists, and academics are generally ignorant of critical pedagogical theory. In particular, the contemporary curriculum reconceptualisation movement has by-passed medical education altogether. Yet, if applied, it could offer a fundamental transformation of curriculum thinking. A curriculum process, in curriculum reconceptualisation terms, is to appreciate differences between curricular approaches in terms of guiding values: a running of the "course" can be both enacted and read as aesthetic, ethical, political, spiritual, philosophical, gendered, historical, economic, instrumental, and so forth. These are the curriculum "texts" (Pinar et al. 1995), understood as ways in which a curriculum is experienced, leading to an identity construction – think of the "making" of a doctor. Thus, the transformations of values perspectives that I have already emphasised as central to the work of the medical humanities (fleshing out skeletal instrumental values to embody the aesthetic, ethical and political for example) are paralleled by the range and quality of curriculum texts. For example, quantities, so beloved of biomedical science, can be reconceived as one species of qualities.

Here, we are faced with two pedagogical ideals that have their roots in 19th-century German education and seem a million miles away from our standard, industrial production-line, instrumental medical training worshipping its central, functional god-term: competency. These ideals are *Wissenschaft* and *Bildung*. They are central to contemporary curriculum reconceptualisation. As Sue Prideaux (2018) explains in her biography of Friedrich Nietzsche: "*Wissenschaft* was the idea of learning as a dynamic process constantly renewed and enriched by scientific research and independent thought" so that learners came to outstrip their teachers and contribute to knowledge as a processional process. *Bildung* describes the process of "the evolution of the scholar himself", a question of identity formation in a complex and uncertain "becoming" rather than an idealised "being".

To drive home this point, Gilles Deleuze and Felix Guattari (2004a, b), in their ground-breaking collaborative work *A Thousand Plateaus*, base their analyses of the human condition on a distinction between a tendency for nomadism or settlement, or for process rather than content. A process identity is constantly in a state of nomadic "becoming", where a content identity focuses upon settled "being". The former is sceptical of capitalism or the gathering of personal worth, where the latter sees identity as an accumulation of value and traits, made stable and fenced against intrusion. The former (process) model cherishes change, mutability, adaptation, and instability, where the latter (content) model cherishes stability, grounding, and permanence. The former leans to socialism or left-wing politics, the latter to conservatism or right-wing politics. Forms of power are integral to pedagogy.

Curriculum reconceptualisation is a good example of a translational phenomenon, introduced in the previous chapter. Here, curriculum content (syllabus) is translated into curriculum process (*currere*). A translational approach to the medical humanities is adopted by Julia Kristeva and colleagues (2020), as described in the previous chapter, and by Marta Arnaldi (2022). They separately outline models of translational medical humanities in which biomedical sciences and arts/ humanities must translate one to the other without loss of identity of each of the players. But, in the process of translation, the value or currency of each is raised (or deepened).

Key here is how the medical humanities, in the guise of productive metaphor, can strengthen the dialogue between biomedical science and the arts/humanities as a process of innovative metaphor creation and the making of meaning.

Working from a linguistic perspective, Arnaldi (ibid.) notes that in medicine patients are "foreign texts that call for translation". The work of the medical humanities is to teach medical students and junior doctors how such translation might work. They must learn to inhabit "the translational imagination" that is "the porous interzone" between the medical and poetic imaginations. Arnaldi refuses the idea of "camps". One must work always with border crossings between camps, just as Kristeva's work illustrates through the process of "settling" refugees and migrants (mainly young Islamic) in French culture without forcing unwanted identity registers. In illness, suggests Arnaldi, echoing Kristeva and colleagues, one's native tongue becomes foreign to oneself. The illness is inexpressible. The patient's language is not simply a text awaiting "reading", as narrative medicine proponents suggest, but is a foreign text awaiting translation. Importantly, as noted, the patient, in becoming a foreigner to herself, is in a vulnerable position of not being able to fully understand the language her body is speaking, albeit native.

While bioscience, drawing on Artificial Intelligence (AI), has mapped all known proteins (200 million of them), it is through taking the translational work of proteins – in their syntheses and subsequent work as "building blocks" – as a metaphor that translational studies can revision the science. For example, the unthinking use of a crude mechanical metaphor such as "building blocks" for bodily matter such as organs or muscle is what we would like to avoid in an aesthetic medicine and medical education. "Building blocks" conjures hard, fixed, and functional units such as the syllabus in pedagogy, but curriculum reconceptualisation asks us to translate from content thinking into process action, so that forming, mutability, and interaction become *currere* – a process of making, or in Deleuze and Guattari's term again, one of "becoming" (action potential) rather than "being" (settled state).

Returning to the Peninsula Medical School curriculum innovation, it is now two decades old and has gone through several deep transformations. In recent years, severe truncations have diluted the original vision of a core and compulsory medical humanities programme, as a process curriculum model gave way to a syllabus-led content model, disappointingly regressing to type. One reason for this was that the original champions of the programme, including myself, have formally retired from the medical school, and driven by a new cohort of management-driven and functional faculty, the two medical schools devolving from Peninsula (Exeter and Plymouth) have not picked up the baton. It is a sobering lesson that complex systems can either expand (translation) or crystallise and collapse (both mistranslation and lost in translation).

Returning to the original, successful innovation from 2002, the process curriculum plan would be based on drawing the aesthetic and ethical potential from the three main pillars of the curriculum: core anatomy and biomedical science, clinical and communication skills, and briefed and de-briefed work-based placements.

The political dimension would be introduced later. This, beyond the traditional, reductionist and instrumental view of biomedical science and clinical and communication skills. Core staff – such as anatomists, physiologists, biochemists, clinical skills practitioners, and psychology of communication teachers – were appointed for their subscription to a broader view that drew on arts, humanities, and qualitative social sciences. They would be regularly briefed about the role of the medical humanities as a binding and productive force across elements of the curriculum, and attend regular, collaborative staff development workshops and conferences to reinforce this.

Staff across the board were encouraged to develop teaching and learning programmes that would stress the aesthetic and ethical aspects of biomedical science. Anatomy and histology (gross and microscopic structures), pathology, physiology, and biochemistry (process), pharmacology (treatments), and epidemiology and statistics (population health) were subsumed under a curriculum structure learned as a spiral principle, where elements are re-visited and deepened on turns of the spiral. This structure, the bigger curriculum spiral, was the human life cycle, from conception to death. The first year of study would be based on "normal" life cycle development, and the second year on "the pathological". These terms were presented as contested, based on the classic text by Georges Canguilhem (1989) *The Normal and the Pathological*.

To aid this, we appointed Visiting Professors in Visual Art, Bioethics, History and Music. These appointments were partly serendipitous. For example, a chance meeting with the artist Christine Borland in Edinburgh at a medical humanities conference led in time to me recommending her as an ideal appointment, for Christine's life's work has been to interpret medical themes in creative visual forms. Another serendipitous appointment was made where a Vice-Dean of my medical school, a clinician but also a musician and composer, met the venerated violinist and leader of the Medici Quartet, the late Paul Robertson, at a recital. Paul had long been interested in arts in health. Such appointments brought with them rich connections and both Christine, Paul and other appointees would be key to our developing and hosting medical humanities conferences and bringing in research grants to support innovative projects.

To offer some brief examples of innovations, we decided to teach anatomy not through traditional cadaver dissection, but as living and surface anatomy learned from live models, from peer examination and from emerging imaging technologies and anatomical illustration innovations such as plastination. After all, unless you were planning on specialising in surgery or pathology, living and surface anatomy would better suit what you would meet in the future in clinics. Students were encouraged to attend a post-mortem if they wanted to see authentic body dissection. This opened the door to arts-related techniques such as life drawing for surface anatomy, drama scenarios for living anatomy, and cutting-edge manipulations of clinical imaging for depth anatomy. Importantly, opportunities such as the post-mortem attendance were paralleled by medical humanities projects such as the visual artist Sue Bleakley making a film about a morgue accompanied by a series of photographs, subsequently shown at several international conferences and galleries.

The point was to educate students into appreciation of the body prior to explanation, and to open debate about ethical issues such as those introduced by the history of dissection. Students would read Michel Foucault on the "birth of the clinic" to appreciate how the masculine medical gaze was historically established by "opening up a few corpses". And let us dwell here for a moment to note again why the medical humanities are key to understanding medicine. Foucault explores and explains first why doctors work in clinics (and how this bestows sovereign power), and second how medical power (focused as the diagnostic gaze) is organised through a masculine gaze derived from dissection. Again, each of these historical conditions for medical practice emerged from a set of conditions of possibility – the clinic resulting from the demise of home visits, shifting control from family to doctor; and the diagnostic gaze resulting from an explosion in anatomical knowledge provided by an underground, technical illegal supply of corpses. In England, the 1752 Murder Act allowed the corpses of executed murderers to be used for dissection. This was followed by the 1832 Anatomy Act that allowed for a regular supply of corpses for the purposes of dissection, particularly for medical students. (In contrast, Chinese medicine would develop along lines uninformed by direct anatomy knowledge, inventing a parallel system of energy fields that bears little relationship to physical anatomy. This was because cadaver inspection and dissection were strictly banned.)

Peninsula students, nearly two centuries on from the Anatomy Act, would learn in a climate in which full dissection of corpses was rejected as unnecessary, serving more as a rite of passage than a learning experience, but this was discussed and debated with students. Indeed, cadaver dissection was seen as a way of inadvertently (mis)educating into insensibility rather than sensibility, shutting down the senses and generating emotional insulation (Bleakley 2016, 2020b). Typical ceremonial rites of passage were by-passed. Again, they would learn surface and living anatomy (the moving body) through work with artists' models, drama and dance students as peers, and actor-patients in clinical skills settings. Our students would attend Gunther von Hagens' "Bodyworld" exhibitions and study his filmed dissections. They had an opportunity to work with both the UK-based pathologist and illustrator who worked with von Hagens on his televised dissection. They would also work with visual artists on "how to look" at objects, or "close noticing" (and its descriptive rhetoric, as *ekphrasis* – how objects are closely examined through a cultivated or aesthetic eye), and they would work in supervised peer formats to study how the body moves, and to correspondingly learn surface anatomy. This would be twinned with opportunities for life drawing using naked models, where we would work with the facilities of a nearby art school. Dermatologists would supervise "body scanning" to "read" the skin; while the bedside examination techniques of auscultation, palpation and percussion were learned in the company of experienced diagnosticians and musicians. How could anyone logically resist the use of the arts in medical education in contexts such as these? Scepticism towards the medical humanities would show a depth of ignorance and stubbornness.

Learning clinical skills presented unique problems because students would learn skills such as resuscitation and inserting catheters in simulated conditions with sophisticated manikins, and this is potentially de-sensitising. The rise of learning through simulation brought a mixture of opportunity and frustration. Opportunity, because the world of simulation was becoming an exciting subject for study through the work of postmodern thinkers such as Jean Baudrillard (1983). Students recognised that their very work process was being reformulated through the experiences of patients whose visions of medicine and surgery were shaped by television medical soap operas, so that their roles as doctors centred on maintaining a "performance". On the other hand, the simulated learning context bore little relationship to live clinical work where transfer of skills was not guaranteed and, at times, frustrated – especially in the sphere of communication. Formulaic communication did not match the highly uncertain contexts of real-life work, where affect is engaged, and emotions can run high. Simulated contexts by-pass affect, the part of human experience that is hard to simulate unless you are an actor.

As noted above, we appointed – as Visiting Professor of Visual Art – an established visual artist, Christine Borland, short-listed for the Turner Prize, to brainstorm how a potentially de-sensitising context could be focused on a novel way, to re-sensitise – or at least make the situation more complex and intense – thus forcing students to pause and ponder, or reflect. She came up with a brilliant insight, typical of artists: move perceptions and values from the instrumental to the aesthetic and political (in this case, gender identity politics) and feelings would follow. First, she noticed that at the heart of the de-sensitising was a gender issue: students were working with the SimMan and SimBaby (male) but there was no SimWoman. (There is, to this day, no credible "disability Sim".) She modelled a SimWoman (see Figure 3.1) from her own body to create the SimFamily, raising the ethical issue of gender bias. She then aestheticised the SimMan by filming it as if it were a Renaissance painting of a dead body that was gradually brought to life through focus on its mechanised steady breathing and opening and closing of the eyes. Students helped and advised in the process. The films were then shown in high-profile galleries nationally for public engagement and placed online as archive.

Students had said that one of the most an-aesthetising or numbing aspects of clinical skills was learning how to communicate "professionally" with patients through formulaic methods, following logical steps. They found that live, work-based experiences regularly confounded any prescriptive and formulaic way that they had been taught to "communicate". They felt that their natural empathy and subsequent care were occluded by blunt, instrumental technique. Christine set up a public engagement exhibition in which she asked the audience to use a stethoscope to find a person talking behind a screen (several recorded messages by students were fed into hidden speakers). Once the message was located, the audience

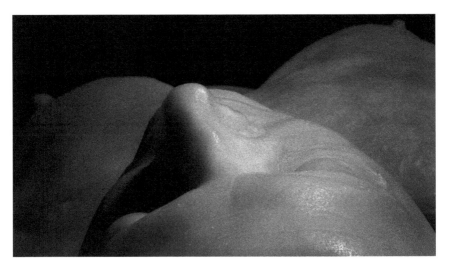

FIGURE 3.1   Christine Borland – still from "SimWoman" video. Image courtesy of
the artist.

would find that it was a medical student talking about how learning "clinical skills" functionally actually served to occlude their natural abilities to communicate and feel for others. Students also worked regularly with actor patients in simulated consultations, and these sessions were turned into reflective conversations about patient communication and medicine as performance. Discussions and reflections worked centrally with issues of identity and performance, following scripts, improvising, and so forth – treating medicine as drama. Our medical students would again work with drama students from the nearby art school to reflect on medicine as performance, beyond the anatomy lesson. This would be twinned with the most sophisticated simulations of depth anatomy, drawing particularly on extant medical imaging and digital cadaver resources (van Dijck 2005). Importantly, seminars and workshops would flesh out such learning by placing it in cultural and historical contexts drawing on key ethnographies.

Such activities matured across the years, and the aesthetic and ethical dimensions to our undergraduate programme were widened to embrace politics – issues of power and social justice. Just as we were launching our curriculum, Rachel Kaiser (2002) published a ground-breaking and damning critique noting that standard medical education "limits uniqueness, squelches inquisitiveness, and damages one's self-confidence". Kaiser argued that educating medical students to be compassionate and engaged with patients faced a suffocating legacy of male-inspired medical authoritarianism and hierarchy, such that the former ambition could hardly get up for air. It was clear that we would have to be far more proactive in our medical humanities curriculum to effect political change, turning the typical hierarchical medical school experience into a democratic one. We tried with structural innovations such as setting up a students' parliament to give them an authentic voice in the running of the school, including pedagogical issues such as curriculum change. We also insisted on more democratic patient-centred approaches such as insistence on "receiving" a history from a patient, rather than the traditional "taking" a history. Language matters, as we shall see throughout this book. But the key idea we had, written into students' handbooks as a headline, was to educate for tolerance of ambiguity. If you are asking "well, what has this to do with the medical humanities?" there is established research finding that the arts and humanities typically educate for democracy through the central trait of tolerance of ambiguity (Bleakley 2015).

Intolerance of ambiguity is a key characteristic of authoritarian personalities, mindsets, and institutions. Many studies have shown that tolerance of ambiguity decreases throughout a medical school career, suggesting a hardening into authority-led attitudes, and this shows for example in language habits grounded more in the indicative (telling) rather than subjunctive mood (discussing) (ibid.). Moreover, there is a strong literature showing that tolerance of ambiguity is a key product of education in arts and humanities (Slouka 2010). To promise an education into tolerance of ambiguity one must also promise an education through the humanities. This provided an answer to the sceptics who constantly pushed for "hard" evidence that the medical humanities had an effect that could be isolated from other variables and measured. Such measurement is fraught with difficulty (Bleakley 2015, Hancock and Mattick 2020), but we were presented with a unique situation to test this once our first two cohorts had graduated in 2007 and 2008.

In the UK, medicine graduates progress to a Foundation Programme where registration as a doctor follows successful negotiation of Foundation Year 1, while entry into a Specialty programme usually follows Year 2. Peninsula graduates happened to make up half of the cohort in our local Deanery, the other half made up from graduates of other medical schools. We used a validated self-report questionnaire with the question: "How well did your medical school prepare you for …?" covering a set of clinical skills, knowledge, and attitudes, including tolerance of ambiguity. Peninsula graduates consistently and significantly scored higher than other graduates across nearly all areas, but the greatest difference was on self-report of "tolerance of ambiguity" (Bleakley and Brennan 2011). Of course, we recognised the irony that, sceptical of quantitative studies, here we were crowing about a consistent finding across a large cohort as statistical effect. So, in the following graduating cohort, we also gleaned data from qualitative study such as interviews and this confirmed that some "extra dimension" seemed to have been acquired by our students that made them more confident in workplace practice settings so early in their careers (Brennan et al. 2010). We were confident that this extra dimension was the effect of our process curriculum model of the medical humanities: core, compulsory, and assessed. It went beyond "communication skills".

4

THE MEDICAL HUMANITIES

A cure for medical education's ailments?

The values prism

Bottom-line, reductive instrumentalism is fine when we are dealing purely with technical matters, logical progressions, and proof of certainties or facts. Here, we are also dealing solely with information rather than progressing to anything approaching meaning or wisdom. In the confined world of problem-solving – through linear, closed systems such as engineering problems – bottom line instrumentalism, or the functional solution, is the most effective way to go about things. But medicine and medical education, while drawing on both biomedical and social sciences, are generally not linear and closed, but nonlinear, open, adaptive, complex activities. Medicine and medical education are science-using activities that embrace value systems beyond the instrumental. This book argues that the transition from reductive biomedical science to the more complex expression of that science in medical practice and pedagogy, drawing on the qualitative social sciences, arts, and humanities, requires an expressive and often radical shift.

Quantitative outlook is augmented and amplified by qualitative perspectives. Intensity, depth, and breadth are increased in the shift from the complicated linear to the complex nonlinear. More, the key to such a shift is in the language and semiotics of practices, as an intensifying of innovative metaphor count (moving again from mere information, through knowledge, to meaning – and, possibly, wisdom). The media through which this occurs, the values prism that creates the multi-tonal rainbow of values from the monotone of the instrumental, are the medical humanities (see Figures 4.1 and 4.2). It is important to note that the medical humanities side of the equation can also be reductive, and that and expressive biomedical science may then afford meaning to the arts and humanities. Artists such as Christine Borland, discussed in the previous chapter and below, attest to this translation where

DOI: 10.4324/9781003383260-5

they draw on expressive science as inspiration for art. Borland's art advertises dual translation: on the one hand expressive science shaping visual art, and on the other (as discussed in Chapter 3), expressive art bringing life to reductionist science and medical pedagogy (simulation models given "life").

In the previous chapter, I briefly noted how, at Peninsula Medical School, we appointed Christine Borland as Visiting Professor of Visual Art. Here, I continue that account, where Borland put into practice the model outlined above, turning information into meaning. She chose as her focus perhaps the most instrumental, de-sensitising aspect of a medical student's undergraduate career – learning clinical skills through simulation using manikins – and put this through a values prism. The argument for learning invasive skills is well-rehearsed. Medical students cannot be let loose on real patients. They must practice in simulated or virtual contexts before encountering the real. However, such contexts are characteristically counter-productive as they rely on using supposedly hi-fidelity models that in fact are aesthetically deadening. For example, the plastic of the manikin in no way resembles the skin of the human. Despite manikins being programmed to "breathe" and to open and close the eyes and mouth, all of this is far removed from perceptual reality – especially the tactile and olfactory.

Faced with the contradiction of de-sensitisation in an environment in which you really want to educate the senses of medical students, what can be done to flesh out this virtuality? Borland's approach was, as one would expect of an artist, to focus on the aesthetic, on intensifying sense impressions. Specifically, how could aesthetic values be introduced into a scenario in which the aesthetic had been drained, squeezed out, nullified by using sense-draining manikins? How could

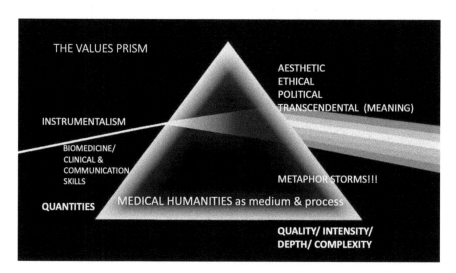

FIGURE 4.1   The medical humanities values prism 1: from the instrumental to a range of values

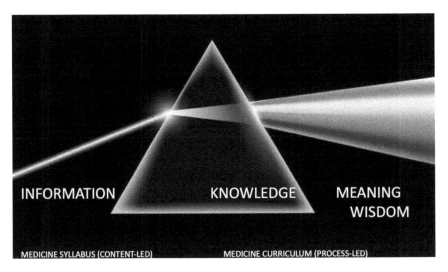

FIGURE 4.2 The medical humanities values prism 2: from information to meaning

the reductive instrumental pass through the prism of the medical humanities to emerge in a different register, qualitatively enhanced and perceptually intensified? More, Borland also noted that a gender-political issue had been dodged, where the SimMan was not complemented by a SimWoman. Her aesthetic intervention would also aim to introduce an affective response into simulation scenarios where feelings had been squeezed out in standard clinical skills simulation scenarios. After all, what would be more intense for students in terms of raising affect than a real "crash scenario" of a person suffering a heart attack, or an emergency context where somebody was bleeding badly, and so forth?

As noted in the previous chapter, Borland aestheticised the SimMan by filming it as if it were a Renaissance painting of a dead body that was gradually brought to life through focus on its mechanised steady breathing and opening and closing of the eyes. The videos she produced must be watched for full effect (https://www. christineborland.com/simbaby-simman-simwoman). The films were produced for public engagement and placed online as archive. Both medical students and clinical skills staff helped and advised in the process and in turn the films afforded an educational resource.

The Newlyn Gallery, Penzance (2007) exhibition of Sim Man (Figure 4.3) notes:

SimMan is the registered name of a life-sized, computer-controlled mannequin designed for use by medical students as a training tool. Equipped with interactive technology that can generate automatic performance feedback, the surrogate human enables the simulation and treatment of various scenarios. This allows students to practise without fear of risk to patients. Through a process of animation, in her video projection SimMan (2007) Borland brings the creature

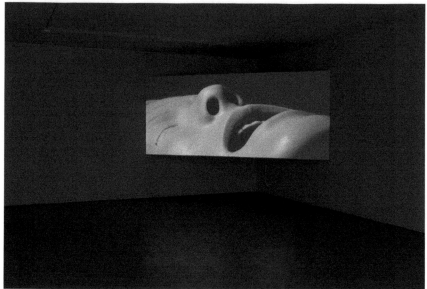

FIGURE 4.3 Christine Borland – still from "SimMan" video. Image courtesy of the artist (https://www.christineborland.com/simbaby-simman-simwoman)

to life, subtly enhancing its simulated functions. Clearly there are benefits to be had from such mechanised learning devices. Yet Borland's unsettling humanisation of the dummy - perhaps alluding to the tragic outcome of Frankenstein's endeavour - raises questions about our increasing reliance on a virtual world, in place of the idiosyncratic and multi-faceted reality of human life.

How we can reveal and restore biomedicine's intrinsic qualities: from instrumentalism to expansive values

Contemporary medicine does lots of wonderful things, and its practitioners are committed. Medical education too has shown evident progress. But more can always be done. Imagine that medicine, reduced to instrumental biomedical certainties, is chronically undernourished. The knock-on effect for patients is an underperforming medicine.

Medicine and medical education, like all bodies, are necessarily ailing, subject to entropy; or show longstanding or chronic symptoms that fail to be addressed. Such symptoms are intimately tied up with the way that medicine is taught and learned, with a chronic lack of attention to process-based pedagogies such as curriculum reconceptualisation considered in the previous chapter. But, in the face of entropy, medicine is committed to healing, to improving quality of life, and to saving lives.

So, let's practice medicine on an ailing medicine – let's address the symptoms that lead to a blunt and sour medicine to move towards a cure that releases a lyrical medicine as a kind of pedagogically-inspired rejuvenation. To do this, we must invoke the medical humanities. The approach taken to the medical humanities in this book is unique. I argue that, like all knowledge structures and institutions, medicine shows chronic symptoms. These symptoms cannot be ignored because they frustrate the development of medicine through lag in medical education. It is the medical humanities that can act as the intervention, tonic and even cure for medicine's contemporary malaise. Offered primarily as a pedagogical approach within medical education, the medical humanities afford a complex, multifaceted medium, akin to psychoanalytic psychotherapy, that can address medicine's chronic symptoms. Again, in a nutshell, who would want a medicine that is drab, stunted, blunt and sour (or instrumental and reductive), rather than a medicine of qualities – an aesthetic and ethical medicine that shines, and engages structures of power with equity and equality in mind? The key intervention in this therapeutic strategy is to *radically raise the innovative metaphor count* in medical and medical education praxes. This is not just about increasing quantity, because metaphors can be slack, crystallised, and over-used, blunt, or plain uninteresting. As the descriptor "innovative" implies, it is the quality of metaphor in the count that matters – new, productive metaphors must be coined, making us think again about familiar situations and allowing us to creatively navigate the new.

One of Freud's major clinical insights was that whatever is actively repressed in the psyche, and then goes unconscious, can return in a distorted form. A repressed memory from childhood of a traumatic incident, for example, can return as a neurosis – a persistent anxiety, a phobia or fear. So too, medicine's repressed matter can return in a distorted form – as symptom. What then is this "repressed matter" and just what are the key symptoms that medicine exhibits, that may be treated through the various media of the "medical humanities"? In this model, the medical humanities do not compensate for biomedical science, acting as corrective (the "dose" effect); nor do they act as supplement or light relief from an overdose of biomedical science. Rather, the medical humanities act in a proactive rather than reactive role – as therapeutic media *through which medicine's intrinsic qualities can be revealed and restored.* Here, the medical humanities act to restore and reveal what biomedicine is – qualitatively rich, metaphorically productive, and imaginative. The medical humanities afford a form of psychodynamic psychotherapy that allows medicine full expression. In short, in terms of values focus, a restricted, symptomatic medicine is instrumental, where an elaborated medicine that has addressed its key symptoms can be ethically sound, aesthetically rich, politically sensitive, and transcendentally inquisitive. I amplify this argument below, where the medical humanities afford a key composite role, as therapy for a partially ailing medicine and medical education.

The burden of reductive instrumentalism

Imagine that your doctor or healthcare team hung a message above the door of the consulting room or clinic that said: "Welcome to a blunt and sour medicine that is dull, insensitive, uninspired, ugly, unimaginative, flat, ungracious, cold, clumsy, tiresome, numbing and restricted". Would you want to walk through the door and submit to such promises? Of course not. Surely, we crave a medicine that is engaging, inspiring, welcoming, warm, elegant, beautiful, imaginative, animated, dignified, sensitive, graceful, distinctive, passionate, expressive, and expansive? We might call this a "lyrical medicine" (Bleakley and Neilson 2021), in contrast to the blunt and sour medicine first described. Of course, I am polarising terms for effect, as a rhetorical strategy. But you get the point. Here is a plea for an aesthetic medicine. (By "aesthetic" I mean the opposite of what is an-aesthetic or dulling; returning to the root of the word meaning "sense impressions", the aesthetic is whatever sharpens the senses, and if the medical humanities do one thing, they educate the senses for clinical acumen.)

Imagine a situation in the anaesthetic room outside an operating theatre where surgeons and anaesthetists are focused on trying to intubate a patient to the exclusion of nurses who can see that the patient should be rushed to the intensive care unit because the intubation is proving unsuccessful (the patient is "blue"). However, the nurses are afraid to speak out because of the influence of hierarchy, where they perceive themselves as having significantly less power than the surgeons and doctors. The doctors, with their exclusive focus, have become temporarily anaesthetised to the wider context (losing "situational awareness") that is plain to the nurses. Here is a plea for a democratic medicine where teams work as horizontal units encouraging speaking out and exchange, rather than vertical units where voices are silenced and speaking is telling, or monologue, rather than discussion or dialogue (Bleakley et al. 2004, 2013; Bleakley 2013; Bromiley 2015).

Offered primarily as a pedagogical approach within medical education, the medical humanities afford a complex medium, akin to psychodynamic psychotherapy, that can address medicine's chronic symptoms. Imagine that medicine, reduced to instrumental biomedical certainties, is chronically undernourished; while medical education follows in its wake, entranced by instrumental competencies, skills-based learning through simulation, and content-led syllabus leading to curriculum "lumping" and overdose, by-passing the values of process and principles learning. Such a linear approach refuses ambiguity inherent to complex systems. The knock-on effect for patients is an underperforming medicine. This is also a medicine shorn of metaphor. Where such biomedicine has historically objectified patients, in fact it is biomedicine itself that has been objectified, shorn of its aesthetic, and reduced to functionality.

What then is the "repressed matter" of medical education and just what are the key symptoms that medicine exhibits, that may be treated through the various media of the medical humanities? I recognise that medicine and medical education suffer globally from structural issues such as lack of financing and chronic shortages of doctors, nurses, and paramedics, but there are also self-inflicted insults to address that seem to remain out of consciousness, as below:

1 Intolerance of ambiguity
  Medicine's inherent ambiguity is repressed through a pretence to certainty (Bleakley, Bligh and Browne 2011) (the ethical imperative).
2 Resistance to democratic habits
  Medicine's potential democracy – known to be the key to reducing medical and surgical error through poor teamwork and taken as the fundamental caring atti-tude of "patient-centredness" – is constantly undermined through regression to hierarchies and control methods (the political imperative). This includes use of authoritative rather than facilitative language (Bleakley 2014). The key factor in authoritarianism is intolerance of ambiguity.
3 Unintended production of insensibility
  Medical education has an unintended consequence of producing insensibil-ity and insensitivity (largely through emotional insulation shown in empathy decline and growing cynicism). High levels of sensibility are demanded for "close noticing" in diagnostic work (the aesthetic imperative) (Bleakley 2020b) and high levels of sensitivity are required for patient-centredness and authentic inter-professional clinical teamwork (Bleakley 2014).
4 Lack of psychotherapeutic acumen
  Medical education fails to instil adequate psychotherapeutic capability for self-help and support of others, adding to a growing tally of doctors who burn out early, or suffer from anxiety, depression, and suicidal ideation (Peterkin and Bleakley 2017).

We can promote "thinking otherwise" about medicine and medical education as "thinking with" the medical humanities – as a "second stimulus" to conventional biomedicine and clinical/communication skills, following a Vygotskian pedagogy. In problem-solving situations with children, where the child gets stuck with a situ-ation, Vygotsky would introduce new material (a second stimulus), changing the context for thinking, and this would often initiate a new line of problem-solving. This works for adults too. Here is a startling example. As I write, the Russian inva-sion of Ukraine has escalated into the Russians engaging in months of deadly long-range missile strikes that have killed numerous civilians. Up to now, the Ukrainians have relied on centralised systems to track and bring down the Russian drones, leaving the public paralysed and unable to act. As a second stimulus, somebody threw into the mix the fact that most adult Ukrainians carry mobile phones with built-in GPS tracker and compass. This capacity can be mobilised, through a sim-ple phone app, where the user points the device in the direction of the incoming drone and press a single button to alert the military who can then bring down the drone. A passive victim status is then transformed into an active intervention in a "web-centric war" (Sabbagh 2022). This works well because the drone's Achilles' heel is that they are spotted easily even at night because they emit a distinctive lawnmower or motorbike engine noise and have a relatively slow cruising speed.

By way of illustration: case studies in the medical humanities from medical education

The Artificial Intelligence (AI) company DeepMind, owned by Google parent Alphabet, has mapped all known proteins (in all 200 million). This will have a major knock-on effect on medicine. Interventional cardiologists can place stents in radically narrowed arteries, something that would have been inconceivable a short while back. Yet an oncologist still sits face-to-face with a patient in distress to break bad news: "I'm sorry but your cancer has spread to the bones and there is nothing more that we can do in the way of treatment other than palliative care". The patient (a woman) doesn't know how to cope with the news. The doctor (a man) – aware of potentially inappropriate behaviour – refrains from giving her a hug, sticking to prescriptive and slightly mechanical consolations. There is an unsettling, slightly cold, instrumentalism at work. The atmosphere is putty-like – clogged, thick, insensible, slightly sour. In contrast, the interventional cardiologist talks the patient through the stent insertion, describing every step and working seamlessly with his nursing team, while a trainee watches and is expertly instructed. Conversation flows across team members and with the patient, who is reassured and informed at every step. While fundamentally an engineering process, the cardiologist turns the procedure into a smooth and buoyant performance, displaying an art of medicine and not just going through the motions of a functional task. There is an aesthetic at work as well as an act of care.

In a medical humanities programme that extends over a whole year, taken by every 4th year medical student at one of the medical schools at which I still do some part-time work (I am retired from full-time work, my day job now being writing books such as the one you are reading now), my group of students joins forces with my wife's group. She is an experienced and successful visual artist with a MA from the London Royal College of Art and teaches a medical humanities module that addresses what the visual arts can do for practising clinical medicine. My group's module concerns communication with patients and other healthcare colleagues as an art – an aesthetic, ethical and political challenge. The module – entitled "Touch/ Don't Touch – the Art of Professional Communication" – considers the dilemma faced by the male oncologist in the example above: do I console, or do I refrain from touch in an era of political correctness and gender sensitivities? What, however, if I am not naturally able to exude warmth and concern to patients, but see my job as more functional? What if I unintentionally fudge communication and can find no way to redress the situation?

Most students, but of course not all, warm to these modules. Two of our long-cherished approaches help: first, we diligently relate the medical humanities back to applied medical issues, practice concerns and patient issues. This might include issues of confidence and self-care – developing an identity as a trainee doctor and acquiring psychotherapeutic expertise. Second, we always ask: how can fundamental biomedical science approaches be reconsidered through the arts, humanities, and qualitative social sciences such that the science shines or is brought up a couple of gears in value? For example, what does it mean to consider the Coronavirus as an electron microscopy image as simultaneously beautiful and harmful, or "awe-full"? Here, aesthetics and ethics are entwined. More, what are the political implications of tracking a global pandemic back to a single wet market in Wuhan, China, where, possibly, a bat had infected an animal that was sold and consumed for meat?

My wife is working with a parallel group, some of whom are interested in using film as a medium for expressing ethical dilemmas in medicine. One student had already completed an engineering degree before studying medicine. He seems on course to become an interventional cardiologist, just like my example above. His parents are British nationals of Indian descent, and he is interested in how to manage his ethnic identity in what is still, perplexingly, a white-dominated culture in UK medicine. But another of his interests floats to the surface – he is a Lego addict. His hobby is making extraordinarily complex working models from Lego. To cut a long story short, as my wife and I work with him, he gets interested in metaphor, expressed in literature and in visual arts, particularly sculpture. This becomes focused on a history of differing views (and accompanying metaphors) of the human heart – as locus of love, spiritual exploration (the heart of Augustine – the student's family, once Hindu, converted to Christianity) and as a mechanical pump (the heart of Harvey and the "discovery" of blood circulation). The latter metaphor grabs him. Why should the heart be reduced to a functional muscle or pump? This resonated with him because his working Lego models on the outside look like purely mechanical or functional toys, while to him they are working sculptures, things of elegance and beauty. He is the creator, lovingly authoring innovative models into being.

Finally, he becomes interested in the idea of entropy and medicine's paradoxical role in relationship to this. As medicine maintains life, so life is running down, inevitably to death. He makes a working Lego model of the heart that parodies the heart of Harvey as a mechanical pump. The model steams away, accompanied by a frenzied heavy metal soundtrack by the band Nine-Inch-Nails. He films this. The model is programmed to gradually run into the ground, advertising entropy and the raising the paradox that medicine in essence is always working against the grain of death. Eventually, the heart runs itself into the ground. The music is distorted, the film ends.

But more, every student writes an essay, drawing on theory, that illustrates their artefact. All work is subsequently assessed according to published criteria (for a 4th year medical student, assessment in the UK is at level 4, or Master's degree standard). This also includes students giving an assessed short presentation of their work (based on Grand Round principles) at a conference organised by the students themselves. Students must pass this module as part of their medicine and surgery degree. In parallel, they also study a compulsory, core and assessed module "Doctor as Teacher" on pedagogy and medical education. This essay gives an opportunity to provide a theoretical frame and rationale in the production of the artefact and its meaning for them as medical students progressing to become junior doctors. Students must then read around their topics. For this student, two strands intertwined. First, he considered some religious and existential issues surrounding impending death. But, importantly, through models of complexity and chaos theory, he looked at the paradoxes of phenomena such as open, adaptive, complex systems (such as the body and the heart) working at the edge of chaos organising themselves spontaneously at higher orders of complexity in the face of tipping into chaos, and in the face of entropy. Stability becomes a moving target. The heart, of course, is the principal attractor in an adaptive system that is constantly re-organising in the face of entropy. And the heart as metaphor serves as an attractor across the arts and humanities – as the locus of love, courage, and spiritual desire.

A wonderfully complex project emerges, illustrating the power of the medical humanities to enlarge understanding and application of biomedical science and clinical medicine issues. While schooled in engineering and mechanical values, and seemingly set on a career as an interventional cardiologist, this student went on to specialise in paediatrics. To his engineering-minded medical tutors, he "softened". In the minds of medical humanities tutors, he "got it".

In parallel with this student's group working primarily with the visual arts, including drawing, painting, film/ video and sculpture, my group was working with both literary and psychotherapeutic issues concerning communication in medicine – with patients and working in clinical teams; but also, in the current climate, looking at how doctors' psychological health can be supported as higher levels of stress, anxiety, depression, suicidal ideation and burnout grip medicine, causing a rash of early retirement and compromised practices. And so, the medical humanities – through topics such as metaphor, language use, semiotics, poetics, communication capabilities and psychotherapeutic acumen (including self- and peer-support) – are mobilised. I ask my group to do some pre-reading – the short story "Mijito" (set in the 1980s) by the American writer Lucia Berlin (2015), readily available.

Here are the notes for the first session:

Q.   Will reading Lucia Berlin's story *Mijito* help me to become a better doctor?

A.   Not in the sense of improving your knowledge of biomedicine, but maybe in terms of the many qualities that you need to practice a humane, caring, and thoughtful medicine.

Why did I choose this story to illustrate the value of the medical humanities? There are many novels, stories and poems that illustrate medical issues and dilemmas. Lucia Berlin's is particularly good because it presents the parallel voices of the patient (a woman immigrant age just 17 from Mexico who moves to be with her boyfriend in California and becomes pregnant as her boyfriend goes to prison) and the experienced healthcare worker (a nurse) in a deprived community setting. The story tells how the young mother finds it impossible to properly look after the child as she is shifted from her boyfriend's sister's home to a hostel, and after she is raped by her boyfriend's brother-in-law. She makes several visits to a health centre where her child undergoes a hernia operation. Finding it difficult to stop the child from crying, she shakes him violently, finally accidentally breaking the child's neck and killing him. The parallel musing of the experienced nurse shows how health inequities and inequalities are simply accepted, but not fully challenged. There is tired acceptance of the status quo.

Issues of health inequity and inequality and abuse are illustrated in vibrant ways through literature. This intensifying of quality is a reminder to medical students of the unintended consequences of their own medical education that refuses aesthetics, ethics and politics downgrading knowledge and wisdom to mere information, also stripping out affect.

The students receive my notes.

"Here are some things that I get from the story":

1 *The clinical importance of "close reading"*
   - In literary studies "close reading" means getting under the skin of a piece of writing, whether prose or poetry, attending to it deeply. In any consultation you want to attend closely to your patient – to observe, notice, listen attentively, pick up cues and clues that will help to frame a diagnosis, choose appropriate tests, or simply support a person who is asking for help.
   - Importantly, how did the story affect you both emotionally and intellectually? What did you feel as you read the story? What issues did it raise? What did it make you think about? How would you characterise your "transference" to the story?
   - Do you think that you have read Lucia Berlin's story closely, or did you just skim? What would help you to read patients closely rather than skim?
2 *Community-based medicine*
   - Most of your clinical education occurs in hospital-based settings ("downstream" or secondary/acute care medicine); yet most health issues are experienced "upstream" in chronic illness in the community (filtered by primary care settings). Does this disjunction matter? Given the need for health education and prevention (informed by epidemiology), and given that the chief health challenges in the future will be fallout from the climate crisis (and subsequent mass immigration) and possible successive waves of viral pandemics such as Covid, why is medical education so focused on secondary, hospital based, acute treatment and not on prevention within the community?
   - While *Mijito* is partly set in a paediatric clinic that also has surgical provision, it is oriented to community healthcare and community issues: of social

justice (inequity and inequality), poverty, immigration, and (in a late section) dis/ability.

- The dis/ability section is troublesome. The nurse tells of her initial prejudices ("crack babies") and how dealing with dis/abled children has taught her to be more open and less judgemental. Lucia Berlin herself had a dis/ability (scoliosis) and was an alcoholic. What education have you received so far about issues of social inclusion and exclusion as these issues affect health (health disparities)?

3 *Characterisation and "voice"*
- A chief literary quality of Lucia Berlin's story is its quality of characterisation and its movement between two key autobiographical voices: that of Amelia, the 17-year-old Mexican immigrant, and the woman who works in the paediatric centre (we never quite know her role or status, but we assume she is a nurse). The latter is based on Lucia Berlin's own experiences as a hospital ward clerk and as a physician's assistant.
- One dimension of the movement between voices is to highlight a contrast between the grounded, anchored, and knowledgeable efficiency of the clinic staff and the "loose", or even "lost", identity of the young immigrant mother. This highlights a distinction between the voice of the (relatively) privileged and that of the under-privileged.
- A second issue of voice is that of gender. In the contexts of both the privileged world (the clinic) and the underprivileged world of the immigrant, there is a gender disparity. The clinic advertises a tacit authority structure where the male surgeons are top of the hierarchy. This is reinforced by the contrast between Dr Rook and his wife, where she takes on the community-based difficult cases where he has the more high-profile surgical tasks. There is both community (Hispanic) patriarchy and institutional medical patriarchy at work. The story is set in the 1990s.

4 *The roles of metaphors*
- The difference between a piece of creative writing and a scientific report is that the former has a high metaphor count, where the latter is instrumental and literal, refusing metaphor. A metaphor is a figure of speech in which a word or phrase is used to refer to a quality that is not literal, but figurative, where this exaggerates or improves the literal: "as right as rain", "a pain in the backside", "bursting with pride". Metaphors are common in medicine as analogies or likenesses, such as fruit metaphors (resemblances): "apple core lesion", "strawberry tongue", "raspberry tongue".
- A high metaphor count enlivens speech and writing but raises the level of ambiguity and uncertainty. Speech high in metaphor tends to be in the subjunctive mood ("possibly", "maybe", "it's open to interpretation", "let's talk about it") rather than the indicative mood ("this is definitely ...", "pass me the notes", "just do it, now").
- Creative writing, especially poetry, is all about metaphor count. Where a typical "case" presented, say, at a Ground Round or on a ward round is clipped,

brief, factual and often couched in technical terms, metaphors are avoided. Does this matter?

- Lucia Berlin's story is packed with vernacular street metaphors such as "crack babies", "my milk is no good", "Fuck a Duck", "it sucks", "get all your shit together"; and the more highbrow "you're a woman now, face it", and "flat affect". How does this help in empathising or otherwise with characters, or understanding how they frame their symptoms? "I shook him to make him be quiet" says Amelia of her baby, unable it seems to distinguish between loving and hurting the baby, whose arms are bruised.

5 *Translation*

- Lucia Berlin's story at one level is all about translations: literal translation between two languages, Spanish and English; and translating across the two social groups: the underprivileged Latino immigrant community and the privileged medical community who are committed to bridging across to their patients. Berlin was fluent in Spanish, having lived for many years in Chile.
- What are the implications of this for a future medicine that is increasingly dealing with immigrants as fallout from wars, conflict, political oppression, disasters, and climate emergencies? How will they be integrated into healthcare systems?
- If you have no Spanish, how did you cope with the constant flow of Spanish words and phrases within the story? Is this not like treating a patient who you do not understand, for linguistic reasons; or who is incoherent or drunk or hallucinating or paranoid etc.; or a child too frightened to talk; or somebody in so much pain that they are incoherent; or a patient who tells you a completely disconnected "story" so that you cannot piece together a "history"; or a patient who is under anaesthetic; and so forth? Isn't medicine all about translation: from technical biomedicine to patient-centred talk in consultations; from academic speak in publications to audience-friendly public outreach?

6 *Institutional patriarchy*

Lucia Berlin cleverly pitches the cultural patriarchy of the Latino community against the institutional patriarchy of the medical culture, creating productive ambiguity (as good writers do). Both Amelia and the unnamed nurse (Berlin's voice) assume subservient roles. The surgeons are assumed to be dominant and slightly arrogant even where they are empathic with the children in their care and civil towards their staff in the clinic. And within the surgical hierarchy, within the couple Drs Rook and Rook, the male surgeon takes on the more stimulating clinical cases while the woman deals with the more troubling social issues: "He somehow manages to get all the surgeries with real insurance like Blue Cross. (While she) Dr Rook gets most of the disabled or totally non-functioning children, but not just because she is a good surgeon. She listens to the families, cares about them, so she gets a lot of referrals" (ibid.: 347).

7 *Burnout*

The nurse says that she has developed a technique of not looking the patients in the eyes otherwise this becomes too stressful. Rather, she looks at the "third eye": "If you look the parent in the eyes you will share it, confirm it, all the fear and exhaustion and pain" (ibid.: 335).

Summary notes (https://medhum.med.nyu.edu/view/16673)

It is a strange and cruel world that Amelia finds herself in. The 17-year-old woman from Mexico who speaks very little English travels to Oakland, California to marry her boyfriend Manolo. Soon after, he is sentenced to 8 years in prison. Amelia is already pregnant. She and her newborn son, Jesus Romero, move in with Manolo's aunt and uncle. Amelia refers to the baby as "mijito" (an affectionate Spanish term for "little son"). He cries constantly and has a hernia that requires repair. But the teenage mother is overwhelmed and frightened. She receives little support.

Amelia and Jesus go to the Oakland Children's Hospital where they meet a cynical but kind nurse who works with a group of 6 paediatric surgeons. Most of the surgical practice consists of Medi-Cal welfare patients and lots of illegal aliens. The nurse encounters crack babies, kids with AIDS, and plenty of disabled children. When the surgeon examines Jesus, he notes bruises on the baby's arms. They are the result of Amelia squeezing him too hard to stifle his incessant crying. Surgery is scheduled but doesn't get done.

Later, the uncle makes sexual advances and, while drunk, rapes Amelia in the bathroom. The aunt insists Amelia and Jesus leave the apartment. She deposits them at a homeless shelter. Amelia spends her days riding buses and her nights at the shelter where she is harassed and robbed. All the while, Jesus cries. Amelia notices his hernia is protruding and she is unable to push it back in place as she was instructed. After office hours, the same nurse evaluates the situation and accompanies them to the emergency room where surgery is performed.

Amelia and Jesus return to the ER. She has been sedated and is staring blankly. Jesus is dead with a broken neck. The nurse from the surgical clinic is at Amelia's side and learns that Jesus was crying in the homeless shelter and keeping others there awake. Amelia shook the infant to try to quell the crying. She didn't know what else to do.

Commentary

From the beginning, the tale is tragic and the fates of Amelia and Jesus are foreshadowed. Human kindness is so sparse. The continuous crying of Jesus punctuates (and haunts) the story. Only the nurse and surgeons seem to truly care about the young mother and her infant. Two very different voices (and viewpoints) share the story - the young mother's and the seasoned nurse's. Both focus on the health and survival of baby Jesus. The nurse has exceptional insight into people and society. Amelia has none. The experience of poverty, immigration, and single parenthood are vividly depicted. In a word, the story is heartbreaking.

Make some notes about your initial responses to the story and come prepared to discuss.

A starting point is: in what ways are the key character in the story, Amelia, represented that are different from the ways she would when presented as a patient case in, say, a Grand Round?

Sue's (my wife's) student narrates a story about breaking hearts that is a breaking of the grip that the primary discourse of a functional, engineering approach to the heart has within medicine. The heart is of course about tenderness – one aches for the oncologist in the example above to literally reach out to the patient breaking the "don't touch" taboo in a natural gesture of empathy and care. Medicine can be emotional. In Berlin's story there is tenderness too, and then, suddenly, tragedy. The young mother kills her baby. The context tells all – poverty, rape, a sense of helplessness and hopelessness with the mother who is not equipped to bring up the child. Here is medicine in another key, far away from Artificial Intelligence mapping proteins or cardiologists placing stents.

My students were asked to consider, after reading the story, the following issues:

- Complexities of translation.
- Tolerance of ambiguity and uncertainty amongst doctors, healthcare workers and patients.
- Use of metaphor as opposed to literal description and why this should matter.
- Critical thinking.
- Appreciation and qualities (aesthetics) rather than quantities. Will the dead child and the confused mother become just statistics?
- Educating for sensibility (using the senses) and sensitivity (understanding, empathy, tolerance).
- Hierarchy within healthcare, including the patient.
- Social justice issues: health inequity and inequality.
- How are healthcare, healthcare funding, social care and the law entwined?

The above issues could be focused and illustrated drawing on a variety of media: film, performance, theatre, music, anthropology, ethnography, as well as, or instead of video and literature. The media are mutable. However, this is not to say that the choice of medium is not important, for each art form, humanities approach, or qualitative social science method has its critical strengths. The point is to re-present biomedical and clinical issues such that they are considered anew or seen in a fresh light that gives deeper insight and understanding. Familiar medical issues are seen, to draw on the poet Emily Dickinson's term, "slant" (slantwise). In this way, medicine is reinvigorated. But note that, where possible, we sail close to scientific biomedicine's concerns. We re-view the science as an art and the application of the science as a concern for the application of humanity. For example, students will be happy to discuss the technical features of paediatric hernia operations all day, but the baby being operated upon is not just a "hernia repair"; the baby is enmeshed in a complex social web of poverty, inequality, crime, immigration, clash of cultures and so forth. The medicine and surgery should be embedded in the wider context of social justice issues for example, as shown above. Further, while hernia repairs are relatively straightforward operations, artistry is involved. How do the members of surgical teams work together? We could divert from the story to discuss the artistry of hernia repairs, the debate about use of mesh vs no mesh interventions and so forth. We translate across science and art, drawing out the best of each approach. We see, in summary, that the medical humanities act as media for translation as they themselves can be translated, where the medical humanities do not act merely as supplement to medicine but provide a set of critical tools to address medicine's criticality. The medical humanities bring medicine to the edge.

The translational medical humanities and metaphor

In the successful examples above, medical humanities conceived as "translational" act to facilitate boundary crossings (Engeström 2008, 2018) between phenomena. Such boundary crossings expand activity systems or create new meanings. The translational medical humanities are then productive of the new rather than reproductive of the known. In this way, medicine (medical culture and practice) and medical education are continuously renewed. This does not promise a Hegelian dialectical movement towards Spirit or an Ideal. Rather, it promises a shedding of old skins, a cutting out of dead wood, a rejection of the habitual as unproductive. Where the Latin root of "translation" – *trans-latio* – means "carried across", this resonates with the root meaning of metaphor – Greek *metapherein* – "to transfer". To transfer across a meaning through the vehicle of metaphor is to explore and expand original meanings through new, deeper, or more intense meanings. A "translation" as replica (an exact rendition) is what might be needed in making sense of conversation across speakers using different languages. But this is the literalising of speech. It is needed when offering instructions for how to use an electrical appliance across several countries. And it is imperative to literalise translation with, say, a patient who finds herself in a situation where her healthcare team do not speak her language, and a medical interpreter is needed.

But when it comes to, say, the medical humanities as translational media for a conversation between biomedical science and an aesthetics of the body, it is imperative that the translation process is expansive, generating meanings. For this, again, metaphor is needed. Deep translation is transformational. Something must be "carried across" (both ways) between the science and the art while the translational media (the medical humanities) are themselves transformed. The fallout from this pedagogic process is metaphor production and a deepening of imagination. The ur-model is poetry in translation, where the translator is poet. But translation too can be defensive, used as a mechanism for deflection or a defence mechanism of the ego. Doctors can refuse translationality by perversely sticking with technical terms that lay patients clearly do not comprehend.

From the above, we can see that metaphor production is core to the medical humanities. Indeed, it might be said that medical humanities work is metaphor production, modulation, and regulation, including the reconceptualising of "tired" metaphors such as "medicine as war" or the "body as machine" as reusable metaphors (Wohlmann 2022). There is no medical humanities programme that does not have the work of metaphor as its mainstay. In parallel, medical students should learn about the role of metaphor in medical work, as indicated in Chapter 1 where I introduced technical medical terms (such as tachypnea for rapid shallow breathing or panting-for-breath; dyspnea for shortness of breath or "air hunger"; and haematemesis for vomiting blood) that work differently in the vernacular as they have poetic veracity or metaphorical impact – a deeper register.

The medical humanities as forms of resistance

The medical humanities are necessarily political. They can participate in two kinds of power – sovereign and capillary. Sovereign power is commonly seen where medicine retains hierarchies and control structures, and can be challenged where democratic structures, such as authentic inter-professional teams, are seen to work better for patient care and safety (Bleakley 2014). Capillary power is not "power over", or authority, but power running through any system that might be harnessed for effects such as resistance to sovereign power. An example of this is "sly civility" resistance (Bhabha 2004) to a dominant discourse of biomedicine characterised by functionalism and instrumentalism. "Sly civility" is a sophisticated, knowing form of resistance to an oppressive dominant discourse that draws on Thoreau's and Ghandi's "civil disobedience" and Franz Fanon's "combat breathing" (Bleakley 2020a). This approach does not simply reject biomedicine for its instrumentalism. In fact, just the opposite – it is restorative. *In the process, and surprisingly, this act of resistance uncovers an aesthetically-, ethically and politically sensitive biomedicine that has been inhibited through formal medical education.*

5

THE MEDICAL HUMANITIES OFFER A PSYCHOTHERAPEUTIC APPROACH TO MEDICINE'S ILLS

Key insults

In the previous chapters, four key insults – as unintended consequences of a medical education – were discussed:

1 Reduction to the instrumental linked to intolerance of ambiguity
2 Education for insensibility
3 Resistance to democratic habits
4 Lack of psychotherapeutic acumen

Here, I flesh out these unintended consequences further, and suggest how the medical humanities specifically educate for tolerance of ambiguity, democratic habits, sensibility, and psychotherapeutic acumen. In this sense, the medical humanities' primary functions are to address medicine's previously unacknowledged symptoms. The body of medicine is suffering, and we tend to turn our backs because medicine itself is arrogant enough to believe that it can deal with its own issues. But its symptoms are largely pedagogical, and medicine has lacked pedagogical sophistication. I will consider each of these primary fault-lines in medicine and medical education in more detail below, continuing and deepening the issues raised in the previous chapters focused on historical contexts for the development of the medical humanities. Here is my credo:

> The more we shift the values register of biomedical science from baseline instrumentalism to embrace aesthetic, ethical, political, and transcendental values, the more we shift from positions of certainty to the realms of uncertainty and ambiguity. In the process we also shift from linear systems thinking to nonlinear,

DOI: 10.4324/9781003383260-6

complex systems thinking. But in this shift to realms of uncertainty, medical education will improve (and then medicine). Our primary media for such transitions (as translations) are the medical humanities.

Challenging reduction to the instrumental, once more

Bioscience has progressed at a staggering rate. Linda Geddes (2022) says: "Artificial intelligence has deciphered the structure of virtually every protein known to science, paving the way for the development of medicines or technologies to tackle global challenges such as famine and pollution". Big visions, yet conversations between doctors and patients, or surgeons and nurses, can be tortuous and befuddled, embedded in historical hierarchies or forms of power grounded in gender and ethnicity. And miscommunications can lead to errors. Despite sophistication in developing forms of democracy (recalling that only half of the world's countries are on paths to democracy), it is puzzling that medicine (aligning with the military, police, fire services, and the law) still prefers authority structures to authentic democratic team collectives.

As previous chapters show, instrumental medicine and medical education favour quantities and facts rather than qualities and debate, linked to a desire for certainty and closure. This runs against the grain of treating medicine and medical education as open, complex, non-linear, dynamic, adaptive systems rather than closed, linear systems. This issue is the subject of the following chapter. Medical education appears to prefer a conservative "will-to-stability" rather than risk, through "spearheads" of innovation (Engeström 2018). This is mirrored in preferences for reducing curriculum process to syllabus content, and for competences and skills-based approaches over capabilities and expertise, as already argued. Meanwhile, assessment comes to drive learning. Learning theory informing medical education is notoriously reluctant to shift from individualistic to collaborative models emphasising distributed cognition (Bleakley 2006). Meanwhile, in medical education, topics such as affective and intuitive-symbolic learning are neatly avoided.

The medical humanities, arts and qualitative social sciences in turn take back seat to the main drivers – statistics, biomedical science grounded in engineering principles, and Bayesian probability models. The irony here is that, historically, medicine has been dominated by two guiding metaphors: the body as machine and medical intervention as war. Since Vesalius in the 16th century, the body has been viewed as a mechanical problem subject to engineering interventions. You can see this most strikingly today in, for example, interventional cardiology. The developments of techniques under this rubric have been extraordinary. But this mechanical view of the body is limited when we take a more holistic view that sees the body as complex dynamic system. Interventional cardiologists may be confused when patients' "both/and" emotional or affective states entangle the cardiologists' mechanical "either-or" interventions.

Medicine as war metaphors have flourished since the British physician Thomas Sydenham said in the mid-17th century: "I attack the enemy within", where

> A murderous array of disease has to be fought against, and the battle is not a battle for the sluggard ... I steadily investigate the disease, I comprehend its character, and I proceed straight ahead, and in full confidence, towards its annihilation.

Such combative metaphors shape a medicine of heroism and confidence in which uncertainty is not to be entertained. This has shaped modern medicine as a masculinised occupation where doctors are leaders of teams arranged hierarchically. These are quantitative-minded arrangements – everyone must be "counted". So, medicine may prefer quantities, but it is shaped historically as a discourse through qualities – guiding metaphors.

Dyre et al. (2022) carried out a scoping review of studies on medical error:

> The purpose of this scoping review was to explore how errors are conceptualized in medical education contexts by examining different error perspectives and practices. ... 79 studies were included. Three overarching perspectives were identified: *'understanding errors')* (n=31), *'avoiding errors'* (n=25), *'learning from errors'* (n=23). Studies that aimed at 'understanding errors' used qualitative methods (19/31, 61.3%) and took place in the clinical setting (19/31, 61.3%), whereas studies that aimed at 'avoiding errors' and 'learning from errors' used quantitative methods ('avoiding errors': 20/25, 80%, and 'learning from errors': 16/23, 69.6%, $p=0.007$) and took place in pre-clinical (14/25, 56%) and simulated settings (10/23, 43.5%), respectively ($p<0.001$). The three perspectives differed significantly in terms of inclusion of educational theory: 'Understanding errors' studies 16.1% (5/31),'avoiding errors' studies 48% (12/25), and 'learning from errors' studies 73.9% (17/23), $p<0.001$. Errors in medical education and clinical practice are defined differently, which makes comparisons difficult. A uniform understanding is not necessarily a goal but improving transparency and clarity of how errors are currently conceptualized may improve our understanding of when, why, and how to use and learn from errors in the future.

Not quite "how to lie with statistics", more an instrumental whitewash. Neither a metaphor nor decent turn of phrase in sight. Note how translation occurs from the given qualitative to the authors' quantitative frame, where "(S)tudies that aimed at 'understanding errors' used qualitative methods (19/31, 61.3%) and took place in the clinical setting (19/31, 61.3%)". There is an impulse to express in numbers, with precision, however facile or unnecessary – a case of statistics rhetoric. Medical education research generally leans towards the instrumental as a guiding value complex, and away from the fuzzier ethical, aesthetic, and political. Even its humanistic leanings are instrumentalised – turned into formulaic skills, where communication skills become codified (see for example Cooper and Frain's *ABC of Clinical Communication*, 2017 – where instrumentalism is celebrated in the title).

Maia Szalavitz (2022) writes in the *New York Times International Edition* (Thursday July 28th): "With the fall of Roe vs Wade, physicians across the United States are struggling to balance the conflicting imperatives of their calling to care with their institutional duty to avoid legal liability, all to the detriment of their patients". Here, then, is an ethical dilemma awash with politics that requires a nuanced or aesthetic approach. We need the qualitative humanities, ethics, arts, and qualitative social sciences (including political discourse) within medicine to address such dilemmas that are all too common for doctors. We need the transcendental also, to understand the entrenched position of fundamentalists and evangelicals on issues such as abortion.

Biomedical science learning presents multiple possibilities for increasing the productive metaphor count and moving from the instrumental to embrace other values. For example, the use of metaphors in neuroscience such as "protoplasmic kisses", "plasticity", "sticky neurons", and "transmission". Look at the history of serendipitous discoveries in science. Pondering on the structure of benzene, in 1865 the German chemist August Kekulé famously drifted off into light sleep and had a vision of a snake biting its own tail (an image from mythology, the ouroboros). He saw that the carbon atoms in benzene would be arranged in a ring, with the hydrogen atoms as appendages. James Watson, working with Francis Crick on the structure of DNA, had a vivid dream of a spiral staircase and this gave him the image of the double helix structure of DNA. Einstein's Theory of Relativity was inspired by a dream in which a herd of cows had strayed and huddled up against an electric fence that a farmer suddenly turned on. While Einstein saw the cows jump back all together in one motion, the farmer saw them jump back one by one as a Mexican wave, giving birth to the idea that light moves as both waves and particles. Niels Bohr saw the structure of the atom in a dream and put faith in his "gut feeling" model. Larry Page dreamed about the entire extant Web downloaded into a few old computers lying around in his house so making all web-based information immediately accessible. He woke up and created Google.

There is the intrinsic beauty of electron microscopy images of, say, the coronavirus, raising the ethical paradox of terrible beauty, or the sublime in nature; the existential dilemma that, as an embryo grows taking on life, so it is on an entropic course inevitably leading to death (and then how speculative literature, such as the novelist Don DeLillo's work, deals with issues such as cryogenesis, or the suspension of death); the development of anxiolytics set against a literary, cinematic and sociological background of everyday middle-class drug dependency (advertised in the novels of Rick Moody, Brett Easton Ellis, and David Foster Wallace for example, as discussed in Chapter 8); and so forth.

Tolerance of ambiguity revisited

There is a fundamental contradiction at the heart of medical practice and medical education that is a product of drip-feeding from a larger cultural world-view – that of personalism or individualism that takes on a masculine form and becomes emboldened or heroic, a dragon-slayer. Medicine of course is the dragon-slayer par excellence, fighting death at every turn in its promises of cure and care. Introduced earlier, in 1784 the philosopher Immanuel Kant wrote an extraordinary manifesto for free thinking, called "An Answer to the Question: What is Enlightenment?" (Schmidt 1996: 58–64). Kant was not alone in questioning the grip that the Church and State institutions had on ordinary people's lives, in particular the way that they thought. Church dogma and State ideologies dictated the patterns of behaviour of people but also allowed for little independence of thought. The very notion of an individual exercising reflection (thinking about thinking) and reflexivity (re-orientating values through thinking about thinking) was alien. Kant began his essay: "*Enlightenment is mankind's exit from its self-incurred immaturity*" (original italicised). By "immaturity" Kant means "the inability to make use of one's own understanding without the guidance of another". Thus, Kant reconfigures earlier models of democracy – particularly the 5th-century Greek experiment – where freedom of thought, discussion and comparison of ideas would be the basis to a mature political system. More, Kant reinforced the notion of an individual "self", a consciousness that could think for itself, critically but with due respect for the thinking of others, laying the ground for what we now refer to as "metacognition" or thinking about thinking.

Kant's project, followed by the trailblazing work of the School of the German Romantics such as Goethe and Schiller, established the notion of an independent, free-thinking self (Wulf 2022). But this also opened a potentially symptomatic avenue of development – the unfettered self as narcissistic and authoritarian, a bullying, self-satisfied, egotistical personality also shaping cultural artefacts. Self was further turned into capital as the "self-help" movement was established, the irony being that "self"-help was achieved on the back of the interventions of others. These interventions were marketed for profit – such as counselling and psychotherapy for the worried well, or self-improvement books and courses. The key factor in the emergence of such manipulated narcissism was the rise of the Protestant-Capitalist movement in America in the 19th century, where extreme capitalism (the making of profit for its own sake) was seen as a virtue that would allow one to become a member of the Elect, gaining direct access to Heaven. Medicine flourished in the guise of such masculine heroism where its capital was also an Elect – a privileged professional group sharing an identity and generating language and dress codes that would exclude outsiders. No wonder that medicine embraced martial metaphors as it framed itself as heroic conqueror, vanquishing death itself. Medical education basked in this hubris and promised "mastery" and "excellence" in every sphere. Control was the byword and ambiguity became the enemy, although medicine was laced with uncertainty. Thus, medicine would live with the contradiction of a history of dragon-slaying (the impulse to control) as it met Medusa, one of the ancient Greek Gorgons, whose head of venomous snakes would only multiply as they were cut off one-by-one by a parade of heroes.

Kant was an unwilling hero where his project eschewed issues of control. Kant's project centres on a metaphor: the developmental stride from ethical and political immaturity as a child to ethical and political maturity as an adult. In the process, or perhaps *as* the process, high tolerance of ambiguity is required to make the leap to embrace democratic habits. Nearly two centuries on from Kant, in the wake of the Holocaust, a group of philosophers and psychologists that became known as the "Frankfurt School" focused on this developmental metaphor as it appealed to the psychoanalytic strain within this community of thinkers, that included the German polymath Theodor Adorno. Posing the question: "what is the fascist personality?", Adorno and colleagues (1950) settled on the descriptor "the authoritarian personality" to describe both a type and a condition that would lead to such atrocities as the Holocaust. The authoritarian is a rigid, dogma-led person who likes to fit into hierarchical structures. More, a central trait of authoritarianism is intolerance of ambiguity. Psychoanalytically, the authoritarian type (and institution) has not developed from an anal stage to a genital stage: from the surety of self-centred rigidity and control to the ambiguity of sharing and collaborating, where sacrifices must be made for the good of the whole – a whole that is democracy.

The intolerance of ambiguity trait of an authoritarian was proposed by Else Frenkel-Brunswick, a co-author of *The Authoritarian Personality*. In the late 1940s, she had theoretically articulated the notion of intolerance of ambiguity and developed a scale that measured intolerance/tolerance of ambiguity (1948, 1949). This scale was to be revised and used widely in undergraduate medical education (Hancock and Mattick 2020). A fault-line then runs through medicine: diagnoses require certitude, yet patients often present in ways that raise ambiguities and uncertainties. Pharmaceuticals promise (and often deliver) in no uncertain terms, and yet their benefits are often mixed with side-effects and uncertain long-term outcomes. Side-effects of pharmaceuticals are treated with drugs that also have side effects. Medical students, in the face of this series of contradictions, must learn to tolerate uncertainty and ambiguity just as their education promises that they will work under conditions of certainty. Intolerance of ambiguity is defined as the perception of ambiguous situations as a threat. It may come as no surprise that surgeons consistently show higher intolerance for ambiguity than psychiatrists. Artists, poets, writers, performers, musicians – all would agree that ambiguity and uncertainty are central to their work. Expressive scientists will say the same. But instrumental scientists will seek certainty, and in medicine, diagnostic certainty is coveted while the reality of clinical work is that it is mired in uncertainty.

Gail Geller and colleagues (Geller 2013; Geller et al. 2021), building on over three decades of studies, reported in a large-scale study of medical students that tolerance of (or for) ambiguity (ToA or TFA) changed across a medical undergraduate programme. They remind readers that TFA is "a personality characteristic in which situations that are novel, complex, or insoluble are perceived as sources of threat". This is important in medicine as those with a low TFA may avoid certain kinds of patients such as the mentally confused. Such doctors have a high need for closure, order more tests, have higher fear of failure or making mistakes, and discomfort with death and grief. They suffer from higher incidence of personal distress because of the tensions associated with the necessary high level of ambiguity found in medicine. Often, as noted, they are surgeons.

Recent studies suggest that TFA dips within the medical school cycle of study (Han et al. 2015), while the presence of the medical humanities in the curriculum is associated with a rise of TFA (Mangione et al. 2018). Geller and colleagues (2021) studied changes in TFA over the course of the undergraduate curriculum, and its relationships with changes in empathy and openness to diversity, key democratic habits. From the literature, Geller and colleagues tested two hypotheses: first, that students who enter medicine with initially (relatively) high levels of TFA will see medicine as a positive challenge in terms of developing the trait of TFA. Situations with high levels of uncertainty will be relished and worked through, rather than avoided. In contrast, another group of students will enter medicine with relatively low TFA, and they will avoid stressful situations of uncertainty and may develop even lower levels of TFA. What the study showed confounded expectations. Students with higher TFA on entry lost on scores of TFA, where students with lower TFA on entry gained over the period of medical school study. Not surprisingly, increases in TFA scores also correlated positively with increases in empathy and openness to diversity. The authors conclude that the introduction of medical humanities components within the curriculum could help to develop higher levels of TFA, and/or stem TFA decline.

What doctors don't do well

Friedrich Nietzsche lived from 1844 to 1900, suffering from debilitating mental illness later in life. He died probably from a combination of frontotemporal dementia and advanced syphilis. Reading Sue Prideaux's (2018) biography of Nietzsche, the philosopher and aphorist a sick man all his life, one is struck by how hit-and-miss medical treatments were at the time where medicine could be said to do more harm than good. It is only in the past 60 years that we can confidently say that medical interventions provide more benefit than harm. This would apparently be advertised by the increase in longevity rates in higher income countries. However, this is not in itself a good measure of the power of medical interventions, as longevity may be more related to styles of life – social and cultural factors of prevention of disease such as sanitation and diet. Also, as David Haslam (2022) suggests, as one advanced treatment serves to cure or provide relief, thus offering greater longevity, so that opens the door to other possible debilitating conditions of old age such as dementia. On the back of an overall wave of success for medicine, one might imagine that medical education is brimming with confidence and great ideas about how medical students become doctors and how junior doctors gain success within specialties or as generalists. But this, sadly, is not the case. Worse, the reasons why have been overlooked by medical education cultures.

Before I launch into a further wave of critique of medical education's failings, indeed illnesses, *it is very important to say that medicine's symptoms can be explained partly (probably around a half of the root cause) by structural problems such as lack of resources.* For example, in the UK, years of underfunding and undercutting by successive Tory governments have led to what many are seeing as the greatest crisis in National Health Service (NHS) history at the time of writing (2022). There are simply not enough resources to meet patient demand in a changing demographic of greater numbers of elderly patients with multiple chronic conditions. Lack of attention to building new hospitals and expanding medical schools (who rely on hospitals for work-based learning experience) has led to a critical shortfall in the number of medical students being recruited, despite the 3:1 ratio of school leavers applying for medicine and those who are accepted. The situation is exacerbated by many junior doctors seeking work particularly in Australia and New Zealand and then choosing to remain in those countries where pay and work conditions are so much better than in the UK. Brexit has created problems for employment particularly of nursing and care staff, cutting off previously reliable recruitment sources from European countries. Many doctors are retiring early, and many women doctors are choosing to work part-time. Pressures on social care for the elderly means that patients cannot be released from hospital to free up beds because there are no places in the community for them.

Graduates from medical school and fast-learning junior doctors are predictably technically proficient as they move through their careers. Medicine, however, has a "non-technical" face that provides healing qualities, where good relationships are built with patients. It is only in relatively recent years that patient safety research has pointed to high, and avoidable, numbers of medical and surgical errors. Many of these are grounded in poor intra- and inter-team communication (Bleakley 2014). I spent a decade intensively researching this area and know first-hand how important it is for clinical teams to work democratically. This improves patient safety and clinical outcomes, as well as work satisfaction. "Team" itself acts as metaphor – sometimes constructive, often obfuscating and even destructive, where a "team" may be an ad hoc group of individuals thrown together for an occasion (West and Lyubovnikova 2013).

Despite medical education's best efforts to ramp up learning of productive communication, it remains the case that in general doctors tend to communicate poorly with patients, for example interrupting patients on average only 11 seconds into the consultation (Ospina et al. 2018). Doctors and surgeons also communicate poorly within clinical teams, preferring directive ("this is"), indicative styles rather than conversational styles relying on use of the subjunctive mood ("possibly", "maybe") (Bleakley, Allard and Hobbs 2013). Poor communication with patients can be linked with the phenomena of empathy decline and growing cynicism that can set in as early as the 4th year of medical school, as noted earlier. This runs parallel to students learning objectification of patients (treating patients as diseases and symptoms rather than as persons). Much-vaunted "patient-centredness" and "inter-professional teams" are far from commonplace.

In parallel, as discussed above, we know from research that medical students show relatively high levels of intolerance of ambiguity. They crave certainty in a world that demands tolerance of uncertainty. (Voltaire said: "Doubt is not a pleasant state of mind, but certainty is absurd". Medical students would also benefit from a short introduction to Nietzsche's aphorisms: "There are no facts, only interpretations"). Intolerance of ambiguity is a central component of a personality style that is authoritarian, preferring control, order, and hierarchy. (Medical students would further benefit from a brief introduction to the post-WWII text *The Authoritarian Personality* in which Theodore Adorno and colleagues set out the psychology of the Fascist personality in an attempt to grasp the terror of the Holocaust, as noted above; also Martha Nussbaum and others argue that the humanities provide the best media for education into democratic habits that resist the lure of authoritarianism, while Mark Slouka suggests that "The humanities are a superb delivery mechanism for what we might call democratic values", because they "grow uncertainty", and Claude Lefort says: "Democracy is a form of society in which persons consent to live under the stress of uncertainty".) As the psychologist Jerome Bruner points out: "To be in the subjunctive is to be trafficking in human possibilities rather than in settled certainties". Language is key – the authoritative and didactic indicative mood is preferred to the subjunctive because the doctor wants certainty. But medicine is all about tolerating uncertainty and ambiguity.

In a psychoanalytic reading – and I will show how medical educations symptoms may best be treated by a psychoanalytic or psychodynamic approach – the English doctor and analyst Donald Winnicott suggested that authority-led persons (and we can extend this to institutions such as medicine) may never develop from an anal stage to a genital stage. Freud characterised the anal stage (centred on toilet training) as one of learning how to frustrate the desire to control by treating play as an opportunity to learn collaboration (genitality). If one gets stuck in anality, then control is the way one expresses oneself and hierarchies are adopted as the norm. Democracies, where eros is shared, are difficult to adapt to. Medical culture - masculine, heroic and hierarchical - has long been stuck in the anal stage of development, finding it difficult to progress to genuine democracy, shared affect, and life-affirming eros. "Adult play" is needed, says Winnicott, to progress to the genital stage and this can be framed as psychotherapy, and, I am suggesting here, as the medical humanities in medical education. The key lesson here is how to identify positively and empathically with the "Other". In crude terms, and literalising for effect, unresolved toilet training leads to shitty behaviour. As Dr Parsa Salehi (2016), then at Yale, says: "(The) hierarchical construct in medicine is the single most important ethical challenge facing medical education today".

Iatrogenesis, or unintentional harm produced by medical intervention, has been recast in recent years as a "patient safety" issue. It was only when numbers (quantities) were trotted out that were best guesses at the number of people who were harmed or died because of medical and surgical error that medicine sat up and took notice. Medical error was a taboo area. Even during litigation, doctors would never admit personal responsibility unless this was proven in court or settled out of court. When the numbers were widely circulated, qualitative responses set in. On the one hand rationalisations and outright denials by the medical culture, and on the other, a culture of whistleblowing and admission developed where patient safety education followed.

In a nutshell, most medical and surgical errors are systems-based rather than individual. This means that a complex system was not understood, or a linear process was habitually followed without appreciation of being situated as an actor in a complex system, leading to a variety of avoidable mistakes. Typically, the complex system that was avoided was a communication network within a clinical team, or across several teams, where "boundary crossing" (Engeström 2008, 2018) was poor. Surgeons would not communicate effectively with nurses due to hierarchical norms; ward teams would not communicate with surgical teams and vice-versa, leading to issues such as potential wrong-side or wrong-site surgery. Senior doctors would not listen to junior doctors. Protocols were ignored so that central line insertions were botched, or wrong drugs were administered. The most basic errors still occur time after time in general practice consultations where doctors interrupt the patient before the patient's account is complete, and/or, patients do not get out the full story of their complaints or focus on the minor where the major remains unspoken. Patients accept prescriptions without full awareness of their side effects, or of other choices, and so forth. In a nutshell, modern medicine does great things, but where medicine promises healing and safety ("first, do no harm") it displays unacceptably high rates of iatrogenesis largely based in systemic communication errors. This is grounded in refusal of democracy.

While doctors cannot afford to be over-generous with their time, they are over-generous with their diagnoses and suggested treatments. There is, simply, too much medicine (see the BMJ's "too much medicine" initiative – bmj.com). Certainly, medicine prescribes too many drugs and fails to adequately weigh this against the harm that can be produced by side-effects of pharmaceuticals.

A systematic education into insensibility

One of medical education's major fault-lines is an unintended education for insensibility in the face of a desire to increase the sensibility of medical students. This can be described as a "compulsory mis-education" to draw on Paul Goodman's (1966) term introduced earlier, first used to describe schooling as a means of social control (interpellation into an ideological apparatus) rather than an opening of minds and sensibilities. I have devoted a book to this topic as applied to medical education (Bleakley 2020b) and will not labour it here. In summary, medical education sets out to tune the senses of medical students, but, by default, poor design, and unthinking practice, achieves the opposite – of de-sensitising students. A de-sensitising, rather than an education of close noticing, can be thought of as an-aesthetising, a dulling of the senses and then a stripping away of aesthetic value. Of course, no decent medical educator wants to compromise the education of medical students' sensibilities. In particular, the development of the senses is essential in bedside diagnostic medicine and face-to-face clinical encounters of the kind that General Practitioners meet day in and day out. There are six main ways in which a compulsory mis-education of the senses occurs:

1 Over-determined emotional insulation.
2 Learning anatomy through cadaver dissection.
3 Learning clinical and communication skills through simulation.
4 Lack of bedside "hands-on" practice in work placements.
5 Lack of self-care associated with poor psychotherapeutic acumen.
6 Sensibility capital of students is appropriated by senior doctors as an aspect of traditions of hierarchy (this is the content of Chapter 7).

Over-determined emotional insulation in the realm of the abject

Medical educators in clinical contexts are aware that students can be overwhelmed by the intensity of work placements, suddenly meeting disease, infirmity, compromised bodies and minds, tortured souls, death, grief, and so forth head on under conditions of scarcity of resources. This is the realm of the "abject" – the perception of maximum intensities of suffering. Of course, students also meet, and can celebrate, healing, positive outcomes for treatments, grateful patients and families, breakthroughs in communication and so forth. Aware of the intensity of the switch from classroom and simulation scenarios to clinical realities, medical students learn what psychologists call "emotional insulation" very quickly. Again, this shows in empathy decline and growing cynicism. It is a way to protect the body and mind in the face of huge shifts in affect and potential over-identification with suffering.

Learning anatomy through cadaver dissection

Many medical students globally will already have suffered insult to the senses and to affect where they learn anatomy through cadaver dissection and prosection. Here, the abject is faced in different ways to clinical encounters, while the cadaver is in danger of being wholly objectified, as a medium for learning anatomy rather than as once a living, breathing person. Medical schools are generally careful to honour cadaver donations, but this is meagre in comparison with the reality of the dissection room, where the insult of preservation chemicals such as formaldehyde overwhelms the senses. Second, the preserved cadaver has already become a simulacrum of the actual body.

Several prior questions may be raised about anatomy in the medical school curriculum. Do medical students need depth anatomy unless they are going on to specialise in surgery, radiology, or pathology? What most students will need is some knowledge of surface and living anatomy. It is a truism that cadaver dissection is a rite of passage, but, like white coats has this ritual seen its day? An alternative to learning anatomy through dissection is to attend an autopsy. Here, the cadaver is fresh and more revealing of living anatomical reality. The drawback is that students do not get hands-on experience and that only a handful at a time can be accommodated at a post-mortem. Virtual screening of a post-mortem does not really help where it returns learning to the realm of the simulacrum.

Learning clinical and communication skills through simulation

A third problem with clinical learning that invited an education into insensibility is that clinical and communication skills are first learned in simulated contexts, with simulation models as we have seen from previous chapters (albeit "bells-and-whistles", as in use of sophisticated manikins such as SimMan), and actor patients playing into the role of the sick patient. Here, the senses are confused, dampened, or side-lined. The "flesh" of Sim Man is not the flesh of the human (plus, the Sim Man is a white male - see chapter 4); and the scripted acting-in-to-role of simulated patients is not the same as the ambiguous acting-out of real patients. In such contexts, students seek the opposite of emotional insulation, desperate, but unable, to engage feelings in highly coded contexts stripped of sense.

Lack of bedside "hands-on" practice in work placements

So, the medical student craves "hands on" experience of bedside or primary care clinic medicine. But here, as testing and scanning come to replace hands-on auscultation, palpation, and percussion, so clinical medicine becomes more about looking at charts, computer screens, images, and test results. The senses are mediated by information, where knowledge and wisdom are shelved or lost and there is a danger that the patient becomes objectified, turned to data as a blunt instrumentalism shapes the medical encounter. Inevitably, as at-a-distance testing and imaging becomes more sophisticated, hands-on medicine fades. How then will the senses be tuned? If I am right, that a typical medical education inadvertently produces insensibility rather than educating for sensibility, a dulling rather than a sharpening of the senses, then we must track the conditions of possibility under which such a miseducation occurs. And then we must intervene. Here, we can draw on the resources of the medical humanities as diagnostic instrument, therapeutic medium and theoretical frame.

Medical students are taught to "see" or use close noticing largely through work-based apprenticeship involving bedside examination. Inspection, followed by auscultation, palpation and percussion were once standard fare in medical education. But, as more sophisticated "hands off" testing through visual imaging has taken over diagnostic work, so the arts of hands-on bedside medicine are fading. This, despite the efforts of supporters such as Abraham Verghese, who has set up at Stanford medical school in California, a compulsory bedside examination course for medical students – the Stanford Medicine 25 – comprising 25 rules for the bedside examination (stanfordmedicine25.stanford.edu). Verghese puts great emphasis upon the ritualistic element of such an examination in reinforcing medical identities.

Lack of self-care associated with poor psychotherapeutic acumen

Medical students should gain psychotherapeutic acumen early in their courses. This is currently missing from global undergraduate medical education. Such acumen will not only support medical students through a gruelling, stressful, and challenging early education, but will also provide a foundation for self-care and peer support through the challenging years of junior doctoring. More, the wider application of a pedagogic-psychotherapeutic model set out here can act to address key aspects of medicine's ills as well as debilitating practices of medical education.

Medicine is plagued by doctors suffering from anxiety, depression, burnout, and suicidal ideation. There is of course a vicious cycle at work here, as doctors feel the strain of a singularly demanding job, so they get ill, drop out of work for a time, or change to part-time work, thus exacerbating the workforce problem. Couple this with structural issues such as chronic underfunding of health care systems, and one can piece together the causes of symptoms within clinical systems. However, something can be done to partly address such symptoms and these interventions are within the purview of the medical humanities as they embrace the qualitative social sciences and inform clinical and communication skills education.

First, medical students can form small, inter-professional "buddy groups" with, say, clinical psychology, dental, physiotherapy and nursing students. Such groups can be facilitated by a staff member or 5th year medical students, but after a while can be run by the group members. Clinical psychology students will be in their postgraduate years and experiencing placements, so they may be natural facilitators for groups. These groups can act in the first instance as support groups, but later can become more therapeutically oriented and sophisticated. Groups can also change personnel. In years 1 and 2, there will not be a great deal of work experience medical students can reflect on in the groups, but year 3 and 4 will offer this.

Second, medical students can be taught co-counselling. This is a democratic method of both learning and practicing therapeutic capabilities (Heron 1975, 2001). A co-counselling partnership is set up between two people where one acts as counsellor and one as client for, say, a half hour session. Roles are then switched. Thirty minutes is then required for debriefing and feedback. The basics of co-counselling can be taught in a relatively short time, and it is safe, even when entering cathartic territory, because the nature of the session is dictated by the person in the client role. An offshoot of learning co-counselling, or of gaining psychotherapeutic acumen generally, is that it increases the capacity for self-care. Given the relatively high rates of anxiety, depression, burnout, and suicide ideation amongst doctors – a result of a combination of structural, educational and personality factors (doctors are driven, high achievers) – it is imperative that forms of psychotherapeutic acumen and self-care are built into undergraduate medical education. Building "resilience" is not enough (Peterkin and Bleakley 2017). Supportive, therapeutic communities and education of psychotherapeutic capabilities beyond "resilience training" are needed.

6

A WILL TO COMPLEXITY

Spearheads-of-innovation versus a will-to-stability

The running argument for the value of the medical humanities to medicine and medical education will be repeated. Medicine and medical education show certain ingrained, historically determined symptoms that work against their full functioning. It is as if medicine and medical education drive with – simultaneously – one foot on the brake and the other on the accelerator. Or, medicine shoots itself in the foot. Such symptoms can be treated through medical humanities interventions. Thus, to recap the argument from previous chapters:

- Medical education promises an education into close noticing or deep use of the senses, but it educates for insensibility (as emotional insulation, learning anatomy through cadaver dissection, learning by simulation, decreasing opportunities for bedside physical examinations in the face of an explosive rise in testing and imaging, and a wilful neglect of self-care).
- Biomedical sciences representation tends to reductionism and instrumental value instead of expressing a full range of values such as the aesthetic, ethical, political, and transcendental.
- Such reductionism sees biomedical sciences and medicine represented as linear process, or problems to be solved. Hence in medical education we have problem-based learning and reduction to competence and skills learning rather than the more expressive and complex capabilities and capacities.
- In turn, the curriculum is reduced to content (syllabus) rather than treated as process.

DOI: 10.4324/9781003383260-7

In this chapter, I address the latter points of treating medical education as a complex, dynamic system where the curriculum is viewed as process. Just what is "complexity" and why is it an important quality rather than a hindrance? Complexity is both a condition of fact and circumstance – an event – and an experience or a way of thinking. Complexity is often described as meta-thinking, or a way of thinking about thinking. It is primarily a way of thinking about doing where activities are situated in complex environments.

Simpler, linear phenomena – such as screwing a nut onto a bolt – require reductive and instrumental actions and explanations. The nut attaching to the bolt is a linear, closed system. The person screwing the nut on to the bolt is a nonlinear, complex system, where dexterity and mood (anger, frustration, a wandering mind) may affect the simple task. Sending a person to the moon is a complicated series of nuts and bolts that speak to each other as a linear, enclosed system. Where humans align with the system, the moon shot will be successful. Any glitches or failures will be mechanical and can be fixed. Ambiguities, uncertainties, fuzziness, sudden disruptions, and so forth cannot be tolerated here. So, complexity does not come into this picture of complicated engineering. The closed, linear system of the car's engine is a different matter from the open, complex system of the driver behind the wheel. The level of unpredictability is such that we need the curbing, closed, linear systems of formal driving regulations and informal courtesies.

Further, while aesthetic (for example, design features of the rocket), ethical (for example, is it right to spend huge amounts of money on space travel when much of the world's population is living in poverty?), and political (for example, countries exerting relative power through the "space race") values enter the picture of sending somebody to the moon, the overriding value system is the instrumental. Technically, things must be right, indeed exact, for both the moon launch and return to be successful. In this sense, sending humans to the moon is primarily a bottom-line scientific, technological achievement. Again, hugely complicated, but not complex. The complexity rests with the bodies, feelings, and minds of the astronauts and the ground crew, especially in an emergency requiring quick thinking or innovative solutions. Thus, while space travel can of course be turned into art after the event, it is not primarily about art and does not need the thinking-with-complexity mindset of the artist, who is concerned about production of ambiguity for effect and an open outcome, rather than reduction of ambiguity for a closed outcome. The artist too is more interested in appreciation of product rather than explanation of its construction.

Both medicine and medical education have elements of linear, closed systems advertising predictability, and nonlinear, complex, open systems advertising uncertainty. Where medicine draws on a high degree of technical efficiency (for example, a blood test), or involves a simple repetitive task (for example, taking a blood sample), then linear approaches are adequate to explain what is going on.

However, once more complex features are introduced (for example, taking a blood sample from a person with a needle phobia, or from a frightened, hyperactive child) then appreciation and explanation of the situation requires complex, nonlinear modelling.

Introducing complexity into medical work and medical education theory and practice introduces uncertainty as a, generally, unwelcome guest. When medical students and doctors work up differential diagnoses, they aim for a definitive diagnosis with a subsequent tailored treatment plan. But, again, human beings are, by definition, nonlinear, open complex systems showing high levels of unpredictability. This leads to an over-diagnosis/over-testing problem in medicine, driven by fear of failure. When flesh meets flesh and voice interacts with voice, when the interactive dance of complex semiotics and non-verbal signs begins, encased in a power differential between doctor and patient, then unpredictability creeps in. Instrumentalism can no longer be trusted as the main frame for explanation, as the healthcare interaction bubbles away, especially when high levels of affect enter the picture. It is precisely because the reductive biomedical stance is at a loss to cope with stretched and frayed human interactions, sometimes at breaking point, that more is needed. It is at this point of realisation that the medical humanities enter – affording perspectives drawn from the arts and humanities that can educate not only the humanity of the doctor, but also the inter-professional exchanges between differing medical and healthcare practitioners within and between clinical teams.

And yet, despite this call for thinking medical practice in terms of complexity, the counter-call of what Yrjö Engeström (2008, 2018) terms the "will-to-stability" is strong, acting as a defence to moving out experimentally to enact "spearheads of innovation". For example, in organisation thinking, complex organisational interactions can be described through metaphors of jigsaws or cogs – images conjuring instrumental efficiency and closed, linear systems. In medical education, despite some strenuous calls to frame medical education in terms of complexity (Bleakley 2010), we have suffered a recent history of decline from "spearheads of innovation" to the safety of a "will-to-stability", primarily through the competence movement. This is characterised by reduction of complex activities such as communication to simplistic "skills", emphasising "training" rather than "education", while assessment of dynamic or labile context-dependent activities is reduced to "entrustable professional activities" (EPAs). Let's face it – even the descriptors are cumbersome, if not ugly.

This kind of medical education by instrumental design is highly satisfying to those who crave the comfort of stability, or show, again, a will-to-stability. But the framework for such technical thinking is flawed if we adopt a complexity approach, that mirrors real life situations. We will see that key to the working of complex systems are "strange attractors" – phenomena such as ideas, artefacts or persons that provide stability without rigidity, inviting progress. These are, again, the spearheads of innovation, resisting a conservative will-to-stability. The historical conditions of possibility for their emergence are a pressing concern for medical education, frustrated by its current conservatism. This is echoed, as we have seen, particularly in valuing curriculum content (syllabus and closed, stable system) over curriculum process (open, dynamic, unstable system) in medical pedagogy. The content of a curriculum can be mapped and remains stable, providing comfort. The process of a curriculum (the verb *currere* means to "run the race", referring to the original Roman chariot racecourse – hence a course of study referring not to syllabus content but the form of the curriculum) opens opportunities for development of medical culture, rather than persistent recourse to the known.

Thinking-with-complexity demands a radical (and not easy) shift in mindset from habitual thinking-with-linearity. Such thinking-with-complexity about health, illness and the human body and mind parallels Deleuze and Guattari's (2004a, b) vision of the "body-without-organs", a body that cannot be partitioned up into separate organ systems – once the favourite template for designers of undergraduate medicine and surgery curricula. Rather, the unique person is a whole that is greater than the sum of its parts, and is a process: the person as "becoming" rather than "being". "Becoming" de-territorialises both fixed identity ("being") and habitual knowledge pathways (stable knowledge).

Where the human body and mind are open, complex, adaptive systems, medicine must enter this dynamic field with an open and not a closed mind. Similarly, where flesh-and-blood medical students and junior doctors are at the heart of medical education, no amount of reductive algorithms, competences, fixed learning objectives and rigid protocols will take away the fact that medicine and medical pedagogies are complex and necessarily located at the edge of chaos, where, kissing chaos, they may re-order at higher levels of complexity.

Complexity is no more a field or territory specialism for the medical humanities than it is for the biomedical sciences. After all, most people's introduction to complexity and chaos theory will be made through science (particularly biology, quantum physics and mathematics). Applications of complexity science are abundant in ecology (the Earth as a living system) and meteorology (weather systems) for example. But it is through the arts, humanities, and qualitative social sciences that complexity theory is probably best illustrated and grasped for novices in the field. This is because these areas deal with qualities rather than quantities, and with uncertainty and ambiguity rather than the logical and certain. In the field of the medical humanities, issues such as serendipity, or fortunate chance, intuition, imagination, and kinds of creativity are regularly considered – topics that are taboo in, for example, evidence-based medicine and, oddly, standard medical education.

Perhaps the key difference between the arts/humanities/qualitative social sciences and biomedical sciences is one of qualities against quantities. In the biomedical sciences, precision and objective fact are cherished (precision too is valued in Minimalism, a key movement in contemporary sculpture), where in the arts and humanities, argument and ambiguity are particularly cherished. But ambiguity and uncertainty are pillars of key approaches to science. For example, Heisenberg's uncertainty principle describes how, at a sub-atomic level, it is impossible to predict the simultaneous position and momentum of a particle.

All known life forms are subject to entropy, or gradual breaking down of such forms, and this suggests that life is fundamentally chaotic, with organisation as a serendipitous and unusual affair. Yet, in complex systems we find an odd behaviour: while maximally complex, open systems (such as the human body) are at the edge of chaos, they can spontaneously reform at higher levels of complexity without falling into chaos. The human mind is a great example of this principle, yet it can just as readily fall into chaos (seen in illnesses such as Alzheimer's and Capgras syndrome). Human minds also suffer from a variety of everyday illusions even when they seem to be at the peak of their potentials. Highly intelligent and sensible specialist doctors can act as if their work were based on principles of closed and linear, rather than open and complex, systems. This is guided by a dominant value system of instrumentalism. In theory, a body or mind can be treated as a closed, linear system or an engineering problem. A knee joint follows a typical anatomy, a migraine a typical course, and a urine infection a typical trajectory. Assumptions can be made about standard treatments: a knee replacement, rest in a dark room, a course of an antibiotic.

Instrumentalism is the bottom line. But humans are more complex than the bottom line – not every knee is the same and the make-up of the human around the knee differs from the over-weight to the dangerously active Alpine skier. The migraine sufferer decides to follow some untested "alternative" medicine advice, while the person suffering from a urine infection advertises a serial case of "non-adherence" and decides not to take the antibiotic treatment (partly because the potential side effect of thrush is a major motivator for non-adherence).

James Hillman (1980: 3) says,

> The clinician takes few cues from the *kline* (bedside). Instead, he reads blood tests. He is trained to see in groups and typings, a taxonomic eye that coordinates with a prescriptive hand dispensing treatment. A person written about in a case report is far less enunciated than one finds in a novel or biography.

Here is the key: complex literature trumps the reductive, type-cast case study when it comes to qualitative detail. The case presentation in medicine demands formulaic presentation methods where information is collapsed, while patient objectification is inevitable. Meanwhile, the high, inventive metaphor count of the patient's lyrical vernacular descriptions are collapsed to instrumental and technical terms. A patient describes "pain in the chest like a hundred burning knives being plunged into me" while the medical student reports the formulaic "central, crushing chest pain". The latter does have some metaphoric quality but fails to capture the flaming insistence and power of the patient's version of events.

Metaphorically-rich description – a form of complexity – does not mean fuzziness. James Hillman (ibid.) suggests: "Instead of measurement, precision". This is good advice for medical diagnostics, as an art. But Hillman (ibid.) suggests that psychologists, psychotherapists, and medics "do not have to become artists and poets, literally" (actually, I wouldn't mind if they did, but I know what Hillman means). Rather "we need but see as if we were (artists and poets). And speak so". Good advice, although again it helps to "speak so" if you do paint or write poetry. Thus, do not fall for abstractions but follow Keats' method of *ekphrasis*: describing precisely the object that is in front of you, or for the doctor, the self-presentation of the patient through attuned sensing. What emotions are involved? And can we describe each patient's feelings accurately without resort to typologies or generalisations ("anger", but what kind of "angry" – sulphuric, boiling, simmering? "Tired" but what kind of tired – lassitude, general malaise, specific loss of energy, triggered by what, relieved by what?) The "complex" or "symptom" presents with specific images. Note them, as a Haiku poet might – with precision and clarity. Now, let us be precise about unmeasurable complexity.

Messy realities: thinking with complexity

In 1998, the Chief Medical Officer (CMO) of England announced that "teamwork will be the route to success". A significant evidence base has since accrued that backs up this claim, showing that effective clinical teamwork reduces patient error, is tied to better clinical outcomes and to improved work satisfaction (Borrill et al. 2013). However, the model that such effective teamwork was based on was grounded in linear thinking, specifically that individual parts of a whole (such as a series of teams or aspects of an organisation) could be seamlessly joined like a jigsaw. Healthcare was configured as a puzzle to be solved, rationally; this, rather than the reality of healthcare that is messy, contradictory, fluid, and complex. The metaphor was inappropriate. The reason why such good outcomes were achieved with teams was that new order clinical teams worked adopting non-hierarchical structures and joined-up thinking (based on briefing and debriefing) as well as generating high tolerance of ambiguity. This was a huge leap forward from older hierarchical team structures that eschewed briefing and debriefing. But the new team thinking itself advertised medicine's seemingly eternal problem of driving with one foot on the accelerator and one on the brake. Instead of embracing complexity thinking, while teamwork became less hierarchical it maintained linear thinking models. The reality must be grasped – again, healthcare work is necessarily complex rather than complicated, nonlinear in the main, and works at the edge of chaos. Without this kind of thinking, healthcare remains dangerously conservative where it resists innovation.

Consider this autoethnographic case study:

Recently, I had a skin melanoma removed close to the ear. The General Practitioner – within the UK's National Health Service (NHS) – had referred me to the hospital Dermatology Department for a carcinoma on the temple. In the process of checking the carcinoma, a senior Dermatology nurse spotted the more serious melanoma. I was booked for surgical removal of the melanoma within the Dermatology Department. A standard biopsy followed the removal, as did removal of stitches at the General Practice. The biopsy, however, showed some residual cancer cells demanding a second surgical procedure with a wider perimeter of excision. This was a trickier operation, as it would invade the cartilage at the tragus of the ear, and I was referred to a Consultant Maxillofacial-Oral surgeon.

In the consultation, this (rather brusque) surgeon said that the surgery would be carried out under general anaesthetic as a sample would be taken from a lymph node to make sure that no cancer cells had strayed. A date was made for the surgery. In the meantime, the dermatology nurse wrote to me to say that she had talked to the surgeon recommending that taking a lymph sample was unnecessary. The operation would then be conducted under local anaesthetic. On the day, a different (extremely attentive and courteous) surgeon carried out the operation, which was successful. I later attended for a follow up appointment. The biopsy showed no stray cells and the wound healed. The treatment was a success.

This linear narrative suggests a straightforward series of joined-up care events with a clear beginning (diagnosis) and end (successful treatment and recovery) (with the guiding metaphor of "the machine", a linear, closed engineering approach). The reality, however, illustrates non-linearity (in this case, complexity) with entangled uncertainties (best described by the metaphor of "living systems") (Plsek and Greenhalgh 2001; Plsek, Sweeney and Griffiths 2002). First, despite a full body examination, the GP had not picked up the more serious melanoma when checking the original carcinoma, the former noticed by the (perhaps more vigilant, but also dermatologically trained) nurse in a full body examination. Second, the area of incision was too conservative, questioning the validity of clinical guidelines for the individual patient. Third, the original consultation with the Maxillofacial-Oral surgeon was unsettling. He had a brusque and overly direct manner, making statements rather than asking questions; and he decided on a course of treatment that the dermatology nurse successfully challenged. The second consultant surgeon in contrast was warm, professional, and engaging. Fourth, when this patient turned up for the initial surgery appointment, after three hours of waiting he was told that a theatre was not available as there was a shortage of staff. The operation was cancelled, and the surgery delayed by over a month. But the surgery finally went ahead and was successful. In short, this was not a linear process, however complicated, but rather a non-linear complex process, a web of associations, practices, artefacts, and communications engaging passions as well as skills and knowledge.

Once a web of associations is set up, both formal and informal, a necessarily intricate and complex set of communications occurs. The qualities of such communications are unpredictable, as are their outcomes. While a dermatological procedure here was guaranteed, both planned and serendipitous ebbs and flows between actors in the complex network occurred that affected the outcome. If the nurse had not intervened, the first consultant may have gone ahead with a far more invasive procedure (involving node examination) than was necessary for the presenting condition. If the operation had not been cancelled, the first surgeon may have carried out the procedure having already lost the patient's confidence at the initial interview. As it was, by chance, the surgeon who carried out the procedure was a far better communicator than the original surgeon and treated his team well. There is no telling if there was any difference between the technical capabilities of the two surgeons, but certainly this patient preferred a surgeon he could talk to comfortably and who guided him through the procedure as he also, expertly, guided his junior through the procedure as a teaching exercise.

And here is the heart of the complexity illustrated through this example – *no one factor was as important as the relationships between factors*. While serendipity played a key role. Focusing on the number and quality of interactions, rather than on discrete linked events, brings alive Mennin's (2010: 20) definition of complexity as "the study of the dynamics, conditions and consequences of interactions". For the one small operation recounted above, four distinct medical communities of practice were involved: the General Practice, the hospital Dermatology and Maxillofacial-Oral Departments, and the Histopathology laboratory. Administrative staff members upheld communication between these communities. In all, the patient attended nine separate appointments and received nine letters and six text messages. Five administrative staff, two General Practitioners, a Practice healthcare assistant, six nurses, one surgical Dermatology doctor, two consultant Maxillofacial-Oral surgeons, two trainee surgeons, an anaesthetist, several Histopathology lab staff, and two hospital porters were involved in the full care cycle (a total of a minimum 25 personnel). This does not include two other patients that the patient chatted with in a recovery department, and members of family and friends who acted as informal carers during this period.

This is a large web of persons with a range of professional and personal attributes, also drawing on several artefacts (paperwork, computers, mobile phones, surgical equipment, dressings, anaesthetics, mild pain medications, car transport, etc.), and employing a complex web of semiotics (signs and symbols) specific to professions or practice activities. Both artefacts and semiotics were key "actors" in this social learning event demanding high levels of collaboration, such webs of activities termed "actor networks" and "activity systems" by contemporary social learning theories that are a key part of the family of complexity models (Bleakley 2014; Mennin 2010).

In healthcare and health professions education, the multiple relationships and connections between people and systems, and the consequences of these, cry out for understanding. To do so requires awareness of the alternatives: are we dealing with a simple problem best understood in isolation and readily fixed through formulaic means; or is the issue more complicated and tangled, yet still open to linear problem-solving? Finally, is the issue one of complexity rather than complicated problems, and then impervious to linear engineering solutions?

Simple and complicated problems, and complex systems

What are the characteristics of, respectively, simple linear, complicated linear and complex systems? How do they differ? Following a recipe is a linear system, requiring no deviation or invention beyond the plan or rules. Sending a rocket to the moon is a complicated process, but not complex, as noted earlier. If it were complex, this would introduce intolerable uncertainties. Every part of the system must be a linear problem to be solved. The process is rational or logical. Raising a child is a complex problem, open-ended, dynamic, and full of unpredictability. Emotions are intimately involved. The process is not dictated by a textbook and requires adaptability or thinking on one's feet. There is a high degree of irrationality and illogic involved. Tuffin (2016) notes that complex systems can be understood but not rationalised.

Even though these are presented as different categories of activities, it is more accurate and useful to think of them as degrees of constraint and conditions that have specific consequences. In other words, linearity can be simple or complex, and complexity can (broadly speaking) be seen as an extreme form of non-linearity where things do not always respond in the same way to the same input, depending on other factors such as context. Maximum complexity can bring you to the edge of chaos without falling into chaos, where spontaneous re-organisation of a system at a higher level of complexity can occur. In human activity, this is perhaps best illustrated by the "aha!" moment of illumination or creative insight, where everything seems to fall together while previously there were loose threads.

Simple, linear problems may require some skills or techniques, but once these are mastered, success is likely. Complicated linear problems multiply up the number of components and potential interactions but maintain the element of rules. There may be entanglement, but not confusion. Complex systems are made up of multiple interconnected elements, with the adaptive capacity to change such that the system (as a whole) learns from experience. The components in the system co-evolve through their relationships with other components. While complex problems can include both simple and complicated subsidiary problems, they cannot be reduced to either because of their inherent non-linearity (Goodwin 1994).

Complex systems are also likely to generate the most potential creativity – in terms of high levels of reformulation in adapting to rapidly changing environmental contexts – as maximum complexity at the edge of chaos (Kauffman 1995). In this context, chaos, with reference to chaos theory (Capra and Luisi 2014; Lorenz 1963), refers to an apparent lack of order in a system that nevertheless obeys laws or rules collectively known as "self-regulation". An example is a weather system or a violent storm at sea. Systems exist on a spectrum ranging from equilibrium to chaos. A system in equilibrium does not have the internal dynamics to enable it to respond to its environment and will extinguish. Systems must adapt. The most productive state to be in is at the edge of chaos, where there is maximum variety and creativity leading to new possibilities (Grassberger 1986).

Imagine a junior doctor on her first placement in a busy hospital Accident and Emergency Department at 2 am. She faces traumatised and irascible patients, impatient colleagues, endless paperwork, and fatigue. She is suturing wounds, breaking bad news, calming an injured child, prescribing, and working to clinical guidelines while also improvising, meeting targets, and attempting to contact an elusive orthopaedic surgeon. This is work at a high level of complexity at the edge of, but not falling into, chaos.

Adaptation is key and the system can spontaneously re-organise at higher levels of complexity. Why this is an issue for the medical humanities is that such work as this junior doctor faces must be *appreciated* (as a complex system) before it is *explained* (the system understood scientifically or mathematically). Rule number 1 is that working in, or living with, the complex system (of which the junior doctor is a part, an Attractor) demands high levels of tolerance of ambiguity or uncertainty. Rule number 2 is that the complex system will not fall into chaos if the doctor responds to it systemically – that is, does not imagine that individuals on their own cause important changes, but rather that transactions and translations between components (including artefacts, instruments, symbols, semiotics, and languages) are key.

The tendency for science- or engineering-minded persons working within complex systems is to "fix" issues that are perceived as "problems" rather than opportunities. Conundrums and contradictions afford opportunities. Those with complexity mindsets will treat such contradictions as resources. An example of such resource-rich complexity (also spontaneously reorganising at higher levels of complexity) is given in the story above, as the seemingly unnecessary addition of a consultant and junior anaesthetist and a junior surgeon to the team in a minor operation, but this expansion of the system (apparently contradictory in terms of use of resources) afforded valuable teaching opportunities, provided a safety net, and made the patient feel comfortable. In contrast, where poor care happens or administrative hiccups occur, the complex system does not expand but crystallises.

Linear systems are not "bad" and non-linear systems "good". We need predictable outcomes and certainty just as we need innovation through unpredictability. The linear is necessary in many contexts (such as feedback systems) and indeed can get very complicated without entering the territory of complexity (as noted, sending humans to the Moon). But the linear will not help us to address, for example, the perpetual problems of non-adherence to prescribed medications and unacceptably high rates of medical and surgical error. Where the system is complex, the solution is necessarily as complex as the problem itself. For example, command-and-control, logics-based, protocols-based, linear, hierarchical, and authority-led management processes are not suitable for most healthcare situations where there is a high level of potentially open-ended decision making, necessary ambiguity concerning potential best practice – including a need for innovation – and a high level of emotional investment. Activities of care are then emergent properties of the interactions between key elements of a system known as "attractors". Typical attractors are clinical teams that have changing personnel but a typical "shape", and patient groups with similar symptom patterns. Sometimes attractors bifurcate to form a "strange attractor" through an innovation – such as the initial emergence of inguinal hernia repairs without mesh that led to clinics specialising in just this technique.

Again, there are occasions where linear input–output approaches work well (e.g., protocols such as administering antibiotics before surgery). However, in complex situations, such as improving operating theatre efficiency, linear approaches are inappropriate. Tuffin (2016) gives an example of how the reduction of anaesthetic drug errors within an operating theatre complex might best be achieved. Top-down, authority-led warnings or guidelines are less efficient than promoting vigilance or "situational awareness" within theatre teams themselves, such as through briefing and debriefing (Allard et al. 2007; Bleakley et al. 2004). This can also eke out "attractor basins" around which potential error may circulate and to which teams can be sensitised. This is of particular importance to the medical humanities because it engages complexity in, for example, inter-professional, fluid team contexts requiring high levels of communication capabilities of the sort that you would normally expect from psychotherapists. Historically, medical education simply has not provided medical students and junior doctors with high enough levels of specialised communication capabilities.

Complexity in health and health professions education research

Complexity is not a research method but a lens and a synthesising structure in which complexity itself is an emergent effect and not a dominant discourse or totalising perspective. Complexity approaches ask for rich, overview descriptions that place value upon the aesthetics of research, such as describing patterns to help understanding of the phenomenon under study. Researchers must decide on appropriate methods and methodologies within the overall structure of a complexity approach.

Given the aims of complexity studies are tolerance of ambiguity rather than instrumental reductionism, appreciation and understanding rather than totalising explanation, and imagination rather than the prosaic, researchers must draw on rich and complex metaphoric language to give rich insight (Brainard and Hunter 2016). Researchers and readers must come to terms with, and savour, the representation of complexity issues through use of metaphors ("strange attractors"), images ("butterfly effect") and tangled notions ("edge of chaos") – in contrast to reductions to linear or simplified explanations ("core concepts", "key factors", "competences", "transferable skills", "entrustable professional activities"). These latter descriptors immediately cry out for the rebuttal: "but what about shifting contexts?" This embraces unknowns such as shifting moods, states of anxiety and exhaustion, re-stimulation of personal trauma on the part of the medical student or doctor as they meet a patient who triggers distress. Here, "adaptation" is key (rather than the more popular "resilience", conjuring more of an engineering and linear approach to complex affect). While complexity models were born in science that can be reductive and instrumental, their appreciation requires an aesthetic and poetic imagination (Bleakley and Neilson 2021).

Representing complexity well

Lingard and colleagues (Lingard et al. 2012: 869) describe a model piece of clinical education research in which they aim to "represent complexity well" in respect to inter-professional clinical practice and education. The rationale for the project was that complex clinical settings are often researched in a piecemeal (linear) fashion that misses the richness of relationships between elements, concentrating rather on elements themselves. Using collaborative practice on a distributed, solid organ transplant team as a model, the research employed a binding perspective of complexity theory, a methodology or "theoretical lens" of activity theory, and embedded methods of ethnographic observation and interviews with key practitioners.

A major finding was that the core transplant team's collaboration with other services – such as pathology, radiology, and cardiology – was not linear and predictable, and often problematic. Further, teams did not necessarily share a "unifying objective" of patient care, but work was formed and patterned dynamically through multiple and contested objectives. "Everyday" collaborative work then remained intricate and not readily explained through linear input–output models.

PBL as a complex issue

Problem-based learning (PBL) was developed in a Western/Northern European cultural context that values self-direction or autonomy and facilitated (non-directive) learning rather than closely directed pedagogies. Such methods may not translate readily across cultures (Bleakley, Bligh and Browne 2011). To explore this, instead of asking "does PBL work in different cultural contexts?" (a linear question with prior assumptions that PBL is a universal method to be applied uncritically), Frambach and colleagues (Frambach, Driessen and van der Vleuten 2014) studied how PBL had been applied in three undergraduate medical schools located across three continents, asking "how might PBL be adapted to work in differing cultural contexts?" (a complex, open-ended question with multiple possibilities). The first level of research, and the most deeply nested, was the data collection *methods*. The researchers triangulated ethnography and interviews within a comparative case study framework. The informing *methodology* was activity theory, part of the portfolio of sociocultural learning theories. The encompassing *metaperspective* was thinking with complexity. These research processes are interdependent and arise amongst one another or are nested rather than being arranged hierarchically or in a linear sequence. Complexity is not the sum of the other research processes but an emergent property of their multiple interactions.

The authors reported contradictions in terms of adopting "purer" forms of PBL, transformations of rules according to local context, and differences in division of labour across the three medical schools. Externalisation factors that challenged "pure" PBL included cultural issues, such as how a "group" is conceived, not losing face with peers, respecting hierarchy and tradition, coping with uncertainty, and integrating achievement and competition. Internalisation factors included variations in forms of self-directed learning, and types of discussion and communication skills. In complexity theory, contradictions are seen as opportunities rather than threats.

Complexity in inter-professional learning and medical school evaluations

Jorm and colleagues (Jorm et al. 2016, Jorm and Roberts 2018) modelled how health professions education research can enact complexity theory, creatively advertising how we "do" complexity. They designed cases, format, and assessment tasks within a complexity framework, with the aim of enabling students to achieve complex inter-professional learning outcomes relevant to future practice. They set expansive learning outcomes rather than specific objectives, including the expectation to integrate and prioritise key contributions from different health professions into a patient management plan. The authors made "emergence" from complex activities the keystone of their study, requiring students to be creative and self-organise their small groups to collaboratively produce a video presentation of a case management plan. Students described emergent negotiation, collaboration, and creation of new collective knowledge as key outcomes of the exercise involving self-organisation.

Jorm and Roberts (ibid.) re-imagined medical school evaluation – leaping from an input–output, closed linear model, where fine-tuning of individual components is the norm – to a holistic grasp of a dynamic, complex, open system with emergent properties. They used the organic metaphor of "medical school as a neuron situated within a complex neural network" to enable medical educators to re-frame the way they think about programme evaluation. Here, interacting systems components within the network include: the health system, evidence-based care, social accountability, research, political oversight of health systems, the university and medical school institution, educational and curriculum design, teachers, and students. They posited that the biggest challenge for medical school evaluation is how to include the communities the medical school is nested in, influences, and is influenced by, in the evaluation process. By doing so, the metaphorical "brain", as an enactive system (Bleakley and Neilson 2021), will create meaning.

Complexity in simulation-based education

Fenwick and Dahlgren (2015) looked at research on simulation-based education to show widespread lack of theory driven research, in particular use of complexity as framework. Simulation is largely seen as pragmatic, requiring a "works" or "doesn't work" either/or mindset common to closed linear systems. Drawing on contemporary social learning theories (Activity Theory and Actor-Network Theory) that advertise thinking with complexity as built-in, Fenwick and Dahlgren assume that learning is embodied, relational and situated in socio-material relations (i.e., takes into consideration the roles of artefacts as key actors). A primary concern for medical educators is how to better prepare students for the unpredictable and dynamic ambiguity of professional practice. Complexity concepts of emergence, attunement, disturbance, and experimentation are key to understanding how simulation-based learning can be reimagined.

This was taken up by Cleland and colleagues (Cleland et al. 2016) who reconceptualised a surgical "boot camp" through a complexity lens, exploring and clarifying the context, uncertainties and learning associated with this example. Using an ethnographic approach, the authors looked at how the bootcamp nested in other systems and the relationships between and within systems, and how passion as well as tolerance of ambiguity and numerous challenges ultimately resulted in associations, practices, artefacts, and communications coming together, to result in bootcamp becoming embedded as part of core surgical training in Scotland.

To these approaches we can add core concepts from social learning and sociomaterial learning theories, as: contradiction (within systems), expansion (of systems), translation (across systems), innovation (in knowledge, skills, and values) and co-construction (of knowledge, skills, and values). We have insisted that a key factor in complexity is the inter-relationship between elements in systems and across systems (rather than the isolated elements, the key concern of linear models). In this respect, complexity theory has a cousin in ecological models of reasoning (including clinical reasoning) (Bleakley 2021; Bleakley and Neilson 2021). This model suggests that clinical reasoning of experts is not a logical, linear process that happens in the head as individual cognition, but is extended (to the environment), and situated (in specific contextual configurations). This kind of reasoning has become known as "enactive", where the configuration of environmental or contextual cues "affords" a decision, or shapes cognition. This is best modelled as a complex adaptive process in which a variety of key attractors interact (for example, doctors, patient, test artefacts such as high-tech imaging equipment, test results, pharmaceuticals, hospital staff, relatives) to form sets of "attractor basins" shaping perceptions, cognitions, moods, and intuitions. Natural historians and ethologists call this complex an *umwelt* (the immediate experienced world), after the work of the biologist Jakob von Uexküll (2010).

Resistance and the desire for reduction and linearity

Health professions education lives with a major contradiction. Biomedical science – as diagnostics (largely testing) and treatment (largely prescribing) – demands reductive and mechanistic thinking. This is focused on explanations through data or information gathering and is intolerant of ambiguity. However, all other aspects of medicine (complexities of clinical work, communication, professionalism) demand high tolerance of ambiguity. Health professions education is filled with similar contradictions (Bleakley 2020b, 2021) that cry out for attention through complexity modelling. For example, medicine integrates linear and reductive science knowledge with complex face-to-face clinical work in which knowledge is applied but feelings and values intervene. Much of the science learned in medical school is never used (but is retained in curricula) (Bleakley 2014; Bleakley, Bligh and Browne 2011). There are more women than men both entering medical school and working in medicine, yet men dominate in senior positions clinically, in management and in medical education (Bleakley 2014; Peterkin and Bleakley 2017). Given these and many other possible examples, why has health professions education not embraced complexity thinking?

Complexity calls forth understandable resistance

In healthcare, we understand that interventions should be based on best available evidence, and it is satisfying when the application of, for example, infection control procedures lead to lowering infection rates, from the Semmelweis era to Covid-19 precautions. But this again reflects a linear, closed system, where input leads to predictable output. In complex systems, where there are many interacting factors and high levels of ambiguity and uncertainty, it is difficult to pick a complexity model off the shelf and apply it quickly and efficiently. Complexity, as we might expect, is a jumble of differing models and ideas whose common factor is lack of linearity. Just as complexity models described complex scenarios, so they are complex to apply and evaluate. This is especially the case in medical education, where pedagogy, essentially a human endeavour and not a technical instrument, persists in upsetting linear planning (Bleakley 2021; Doll et al. 2005; Trueit 2013).

If there were a best linear method of educating medical students, we would have perfected it by now. Further, it could be replicated. But no such blueprint exists because medical education is about ever-shifting, context-dependent qualities. Many have tried, reducing complex curricula processes to content-based syllabi, pedagogy to instruction, learning to observable competences, patients to "problems" to be solved through problem-based learning, diagnostics to formulaic algorithms such as decision trees; and assessment to "objective", "structured" clinical examinations, and so forth. Instrumentalism and technical solutions are sought through the inappropriate framing of medical education as a closed, linear system, where such an education is complex, and process outstrips content. Whatever the level of strain it puts upon us, we must be ingenious in understanding that just as healthcare is complex, so too is health professions education.

It is as important to recognise, and attend to, defences against adopting complexity models as it is to educate in those models. In fact, the first must precede the second. If complexity is neither grasped nor seen to work, then it will be readily ditched as pragmatic healthcare educators return to the safety of closed, linear models rather than embrace innovation (with all its associated risks and uncertainties) (Engeström 2018). We might liken this to climate change denial. Addressing climate change demands that we understand its complex dynamics and grounding in collaborative action. The singular resistance of the individual is an example of burying one's head in the sand. Resistance to complexity theory in medicine may be grounded in an unacknowledged ideology of individualism or autonomy as an historical habit (the lone, heroic doctor), resisting thinking in terms of metaphors such as exchanges, webs, patterns, and collaborations (Bleakley, Bligh and Browne 2011; Glouberman and Zimmerman 2002). Bleakley (2021) sees a power, or political, issue at work here, where lingering hierarchies (in which patterns of medical error are grounded) are being replaced by more democratic structures and habits (grounded in patient-centredness and inter-professionalism). Inevitably, patterns of resistance arise grounded in old habits that frustrate such potential innovation.

Against such resistance to complexity, it is sufficient to know, as Trent (2019) points out, that a failure to model healthcare systems on complexity has led indirectly to unacceptably high rates of medical and surgical error. Systems such as clinical teams fail to be appreciated as parts of wider healthcare systems, particularly numbers of teams interacting around a patient, such that communication breakdowns are common not just within teams (because of the insistence on maintaining hierarchies), but also across teams (failure to appreciate how systems can be built that generate both communication and adaptation rather than stifling them) (Bleakley et al. 2004). Trent (2019) describes this in terms of how feedback is enacted:

> All complex adaptive systems have some form of a feedback mechanism in place to ensure they can reach a level of optimisation organically... When feedback is ignored, the system will quickly spiral out of control and collapse: A cancerous cell ignores the feedback mechanisms that normally would trigger apoptosis. Beta cells in a diabetic person's pancreas ignore the elevated levels of blood glucose... when feedback is ignored, the system collapses. The cancer grows, the blood sugar rises, the patient dies... Health care systems have little to zero feedback mechanisms in place. When they are implemented, there is an almost immediate improvement.

So, who will grasp the nettle of complexity and responsibility for ensuring that feedback mechanisms are developed? Cristancho, Field, and Lingard (2019) claim that complexity is fast becoming a "God term" (an untouchable invocation of something important and mysterious that is immune to critical enquiry) in medical education. However, we question this given the same authors identified only 46 papers describing the use of complexity science in medical education in the period 2000–17. This is a drop in the ocean in comparison to, say, papers on PBL, professionalism, competence frameworks, learning by simulation, work-based learning, curriculum frameworks, and so forth. After two decades, complexity theory simply hasn't got a strong foothold in health professions education. This can be put down to the relative comfort and safety of linear approaches, compared with the high-risk factor in complexity.

The linear tic – a stain on the cloth of complexity

While the literature on use of complexity theory in health professions education research has grown in recent years (Brainard and Hunter 2016; Chandler et al. 2015; Cristancho et al. 2019; Fenwick and Dahlgren 2015; Jorm et al. 2016; Jorm and Roberts 2018; Pinsky 2010) there is an ironic trend – the desire to reduce complexity to instrumental principles echoing linearity. It is like an anchor that prevents us from setting sail or ascending in the basket of the balloon. This is a widespread issue and even the best accounts of complexity seem to seek an anchor of linearity, a safe harbour. For example, the educationalist William Doll (Doll et al. 2005: 171; Trueit 2013) persistently warns against linear restrictions to curriculum such as restrictive pre-set goals (outcomes) that in turn dictate syllabus content and assessment methods. Yet, in the same breath, he calls for a shift "towards a curriculum *rich* in problematics, *recursive* in its nonlinear organisation, *relational* in its structure, and *rigorous* in its application". The four R's suggesting linearity by the back door – a mnemonic or even a formula, rather than an alliterative poetic device that one might expect from Doll (one should never call on alliteration more than three times in a sentence). Similarly, Mennin (2010: 20) echoes Doll's linear summary model, borrowing his terminology, where:

> The core process of complexity, self-organisation, requires a system that is open and far from equilibrium, with ill-defined boundaries and a large number of non-linear interactions involving short-loop feedback… An approach to curriculum based on self-organisation is characterised as rich, recursive, relational and rigorous and it illuminates how a curriculum can be understood as a complex adaptive system.

We saw above that Jorm and Roberts (2018) adopt a four key factors approach (nesting, diversity, self-organisation, and emergent outcomes). Chandler and colleagues (Chandler et al. 2015) move to a five core concepts approach (self-organisation, interaction, emergence, system history, and temporality). Fenwick and Dahlgren (2015) adopt a three-factor approach to learning (as embodied, relational, and situated in social–material relations), and a four-factor framework of complexity (emergence, attunement, disturbance, and experimentation).

We are suspicious of this formulaic reduction amongst authors on complexity that we admire. Is an anchor of linearity again preventing us from setting sail or achieving unencumbered full flight? Once one enters the field of complexity, all kinds of ambiguities, paradoxes, aporias, contradictions, and disturbances arise.

Trying to iron them out systematically (such as reduction to principles or rules of thumb) is largely counterproductive, simply reinforcing that you cannot reduce an open, dynamic, nonlinear complex system to a closed, linear explanation without losing the complexity that identifies the system in the first place.

To research healthcare and health professions education with complexity theory, one must "think with complexity" or have a complexity mindset that itself rationalises linearity as "appropriate for context". Thinking-with-complexity is a metacognition equivalent to critically reflexive practice – being able to reflect on the values that shape one's practices, put these values in the perspective of practices of others, and to shift these values of necessary. Cristancho, Field, and Lingard (2019) ask a pertinent question:

> Do medical education scholars understand that there are multiple legitimate orientations to complexity science, deriving from distinct disciplinary origins, drawing on different metaphors and serving distinct purposes? If we do not understand this, a cascade of potential consequences awaits. We may assume that complexity science is singular in that there is only one way to do it. This assumption may cause us to perceive our way as the 'right' way and to disregard other approaches as illegitimate. However, this perception of illegitimacy may limit our ability to enter into productive dialogue about our complexity science-inspired research.

In short, there are many versions of complexity and systems fit circumstances. One kind of complexity modelling may help to understand how factors interact in the development of skin cancers. Another model may be needed to help us to understand the relationships between health and inequities, and inequalities related to skin colour and ethnicity.

In summary, thinking with complexity is akin to making the leap from explaining and exploring human health and illness through an instrumental, bottom-line biomedical science lens (linear, closed models) as opposed to a fulsome biomedical science that embraces aesthetic, political, ethical, and transcendental values (nonlinear, open, adaptive models). The latter naturally embraces the arts, humanities, and qualitative social sciences as equal partners in cultivation of an imagination of complexity.

Acknowledgement

This chapter was written in collaboration with Professor Jennifer Cleland.

7

THE DISTRIBUTION OF THE SENSIBLE

Welcome to the revolution!

As the previous chapter explored, a first major overhaul of medicine and medical education is to shift from linear, engineering thinking to whole systems thinking (adaptive, complex, aesthetic, self-regulating). A second overhaul is to shift from hierarchies to authentic democracies within medical practice, where patient-centredness and inter-professional teamworking are commonplace. A third overhaul is to create equality of opportunity for public healthcare provision globally. And a fourth is to provide the educational opportunities early in a medical student's career to learn basic psychotherapeutic acumen that will shape self-care and communication with patients and colleagues. These overhauls signal major organisational shifts – evident in patches throughout global medicine and medical education, but not established as the norm. Again, adoption of key aspects of the medical humanities within medical education could stimulate a shift to systems thinking, authentic democratic habits and equity in global public healthcare, as well as psychotherapeutic acumen necessary for the job. What has held up these changes is a series of resistances within medicine and medical education addressed throughout this book. In this chapter I look at resistance constellating around education of the senses. This is embedded in the second overhaul listed above: to shift from hierarchies to authentic democracies. I consider the work of the senses as basic capital within medicine and medical education, open to ownership and distribution/ redistribution according to vested, hierarchical interests. How can we achieve a democratic distribution of sensibility in medical work in the face of historically contingent, embedded hierarchy?

Given the critical importance of using the senses in diagnostic work, one might think that focused education of the senses would be a curriculum priority for

DOI: 10.4324/9781003383260-8

medical education. This is not the case – education of the senses is not meticulously planned but left largely to chance encounters in work-based learning that itself is largely spontaneous. Systematic briefing and de-briefing of work placements are relatively rare, while major learning opportunities such as bedside practice in hospital settings often eschews hands-on opportunities for palpation, auscultation, and percussion – where remote testing is more common (such as blood tests or imaging). Of course, such testing gives more accurate results, but hands-on, immediate gathering of signs and symptoms through the senses affords a wider opportunity – that of making deeper and more intimate contact with the patient. Quoted previously, but worth repeating, as James Hillman (1980: 3) says,

> The clinician takes few cues from the *kline* (bedside). Instead, he reads blood tests. He is trained to see in groups and typings, a taxonomic eye that coordinates with a prescriptive hand dispensing treatment. A person written about in a case report is far less enunciated than one finds in a novel or biography.

I have written at length about education of the senses through the medical humanities (Bleakley 2020b). Here, I will take a different tack that is more about politics and ethics than aesthetics (that literally means 'sense impressions'). In terms of aesthetics, where it is vitally important that medical students are given educational opportunities to extend and intensify clinical uses of the senses, encompassing diagnostic and communication work, we find medical education systematically closing the senses down through three main channels. First, the still common practice of learning anatomy through cadaver dissection can overwhelm the senses rather than sharpening and focusing them. Second, exposure to disease, death, and suffering can of course be overwhelming, and students are encouraged to develop emotional insulation, where natural feelings of empathy, pity, and disgust are suppressed for rational, cognitive responses. This is embedded in a wider cultural effect in medical education that relegates the importance of affect. And third, learning clinical and communication skills through simulation, working with manikins for example, shuts down the senses and feelings for a kind of blank "acting into" the role. All these objections have been widely documented (ibid.) and discussed in previous chapters.

In terms of politics and ethics, in this chapter my focus will be on how the uses and education of the senses can be framed as "capital" that is generated, distributed, withheld, and controlled in the same way that physical capital such as goods or money are manipulated by key interests through power structures. Here, I follow the lead of Jacques Rancière (1991, 1995, 2006a, 2006b, 2010, 2011, 2013), whose work is key to the arguments presented in this chapter. Capital too can be intellectual (for example involving intellectual rights to ideas); bodily (people's physical labour is regularly bought and sold on markets; bodies – mainly women – are trafficked and enslaved largely through the sex trade); transcendental (search for meaning has long been packaged and marketed as product, particularly through

New Age spiritual "growth" programmes); and emotional (feelings are subject to power relationships – at a cultural level vested interests set out to control feelings through dictated conventions such as how a ruling class may set "standards" for the masses; at a personal level of, say, intimacy in a relationship, one partner may come to control the feeling states of another, dictating his or her responses).

Classic liberatory models of power, stemming from Marx's analyses and critique of capitalism as a way of production and distribution of power for vested interest profit, see power as "sovereign". Here, power is evident in concrete exchanges, such as a ruler extracting taxes from the populace, or an employer deciding how much a worker's labour is worth (de-personalising the human as "units" of productivity) and by how much labour should be compensated. However, since the ground-breaking work of Michel Foucault (2020), we now think of power not only as sovereign ("power over"), but also as capillary ("power through"). Foucault's analysis frames power not just as controlling (sovereign) but also as forms of resistance to such control (capillary).

In sovereign power terms, where a patient refuses a prescribed medicine or course of treatment that a doctor feels will help her, the doctor's prescription is a legitimate authority gesture and the patient's refusal is labelled as "noncompliance" (the term is loaded, indicating refusal by patients as a breach of agreement). In capillary power terms, the patient's refusal may be a justified resistance to an unwanted intervention ("I know my body and mind better than you do"). Resistances can be strong and overt (physical, as in combat; politically organised to challenge authority, as in the suffragette movement or anti-racist movements; or overwhelming through numbers as in Ghandi's non-violent protest; or challenging habit, as in the women of warring cities in Aristophanes' *Lysistra* withholding sex from their husbands and lovers as means of persuading the men to end the Peloponnesian War between Greek City States). Or they can be subtle yet penetrating, the latter illustrated by "sly civility" approaches (Bhabha 2004) where resistance is not direct, but by subtle, indirect undermining of authority – a "slant" gesture of power.

Giorgio Agamben (1995) suggests that Foucault goes too far in arguing for capillary power, so that we see capillary power everywhere as a kind of permeating ghost, forgetting that repressive regimes exist that exert sovereign power openly and this must be attended to. Agamben wonders why Foucault's writings never addressed the Holocaust, the most alarming example of a negative sovereign power at work. Jean Baudrillard (1988) suggests that capillary power can become a simulacrum – a copy of a copy where there is no original. Indeed, capillary power can become symptom. A primary example of capillary power is self-control or self-regulation, clearly important in professional activities such as medicine where emotions can be provoked so readily. However, self-regulation, as "self-forming" of identity, can also take twists and turns into symptoms such as narcissism, historically a "dark" marker for physicians as they separate themselves from other healthcare professionals and patients within hierarchies.

We begin to imagine capillary power at work even where there is no concrete evidence of its existence. The most obvious example, following from the self-regulation example above, is one's conscience. This is Freud's superego at work – you might feel guilty for something that has little consequence and is readily forgotten. Is this really "power" at work? It is surely too trivial. Let me give you an example of this ghost power. Driving home late at night, in the dark and with an impending storm, a flash occurred. I mistook a flash of lightning for a speed camera, even though I knew the road well and that no speed cameras existed on that stretch. Power becomes internalised as forms of surveillance, associated with transgression leading to guilt. But these forms are simulacra. "Conscience" here, as Baudrillard describes it, is a tissue of lies, a fabrication. Doctors, physiotherapists, psychotherapists, and others who work with intimate bodily and emotional exposure learn to sublimate inappropriate desire through "professionalism", but how this sublimation is learned and exercised is rarely discussed in medical education, where it is central to the education of psychotherapists as the management of countertransference and counter-resistance.

Embracing both sovereign and capillary power effects, Jacques Rancière describes a range of occasions in which power (politics), ethics and aesthetics interact. His focus is on how power structures and the distribution of power affect how we sense. In the remainder of the chapter, I show how this model can have impact on our understanding of the distribution of power within medical culture, affecting educational quality and opportunity. Here is an example of how the medical humanities' interest in the entanglement of ethics, aesthetics, and politics, away from the purely instrumental focus of the biomedical sciences and clinical/ communication skills, can be of great value in pedagogy, such as curriculum planning.

As André Gorz (2010) points out, capital is not just material, but also immaterial. Knowledge and emotional labour are two kinds of immaterial capital. They are hard for capitalists to commodify and exploit yet they have obvious intrinsic and exchange value (for example in the field of "intellectual property"). In medicine, value is explicit in a doctor's or surgeon's technical knowledge and skill, but also in his or her communication prowess, imagination and creativity, and ability to manage affect or emotional labour. As the medical student becomes a junior doctor, one might think that gaining an identity is the key source of capital gain. The qualified "doctor" becomes a sought-after commodity yet is one that is exploited within the medical community itself.

Jacques Rancière's triquetra knot: aesthetics, politics, and ethics

You will be lucky to hear of medical educationalists who draw on Jacques Rancière's work, although educationalists in general do. Worse, the medical humanities in medical education community do not entertain, and then discuss, his work, while he is revered amongst humanities scholars. Yet Rancière is one of the principal thinkers on relationships between power (politics) and aesthetics, that naturally invokes ethical issues. Where medical education in general has failed to address links between aesthetics and politics, within the field of the medical/health humanities there is a rapidly growing interest in addressing health inequities and inequalities – and social justice issues in general – through two aesthetic channels: a "pedagogy of the oppressed" as proposed by Paulo Freire (1996), and a "theatre of the oppressed" as proposed by Augusto Boal (1991), who was directly influenced by Freire. Such frameworks have been applied globally to medical and healthcare education to help students to develop an appreciation of health inequalities (Ramaswamy and Ramaswamy 2020).

While he does not acknowledge or pursue the idea, Rancière thinks in open systems terms – holistically – rather than in closed, linear engineering terms (see Chapter 6). Central to his work on aesthetics and politics is the notion that cultures can spontaneously reorganise at higher levels of complexity as they engage with the fields of aesthetics (beauty and form) in relationship to power structures. Primarily, for Rancière, shaping a democracy is an act of beauty or form prior to function, requiring a vision. But this "beauty" can be rough-and-ready while artisanal and grounded in the vernacular, or of the people. Rancière traces a rich history of folk arts as opposed to high art, pointing out how the latter typically oppresses the former. I have already pointed out how everyday metaphor-rich vernacular language of the lay public offers a rich aesthetic medium for doctor-patient encounters that is often displaced by technical-medical lingo (as noted, the clinico-technical term *tachypnoea* is equitably translated as "abnormal rapid breathing", but the vernacular is "panting for breath", a wonderful, embodied metaphor). This is an anaesthetising and smoothing of the often sharp or contoured encounter, helpful for the doctor where a long series of intense encounters in a pressing daily schedule cannot be too acute or emotionally demanding.

Significant social change in medical education cannot be achieved without first embracing medical pedagogy as holistic and complex process (*currere*) focused on identity production and culture change, as well as such an education functioning to some extent as a linear system with means-ends structures (such as learning objectives and focused teaching techniques). Such a pedagogical revolution can be both political and aesthetic. Medical students would not be expected to read Rancière or similar authors, but medical educators, including clinicians, should. They would benefit from grasping just how aesthetics and politics are closely bound by also reading *The Aesthetics of Resistance*, a novel by Peter Weiss (2005, 2020). Here, Resistance activists in Nazi Germany (during the rise to power of Hitler) and Fascist Italy (during the Spanish Civil War) learn to give democratic habits gestural form, or to shape their activism as grace under severe pressure (in being pursued, sent to concentration camps, or in combat). Activism gives rise to genres such as "resistance" poetry and music.

In a free-market capitalist economy, where surplus capital is utilised to produce further profit, such profit is typically unfairly redistributed. For example, at the time of writing, in the current global energy crisis exacerbated by the war waged by Russia upon Ukraine, oil and gas prices have risen considerably. But energy companies have ensured that their profits remain high, while dividends are passed on to shareholders (where the companies themselves retain shares in their own businesses). Here, profits are not distributed amongst company workers (except the top level of management) nor are they distributed to consumers through cutting prices.

In the case of company workers, or workers in general, it is not just physical or intellectual labour that is exploited, but also "emotional labour", a term coined by Arlie Hochschild (1983). In any work context, feelings are regulated and managed appropriately and this, in for example the "front end" service industries, is a central part of the job. Famously, in *Being and Nothingness* Jean Paul Sartre (2003) describes an over-eager waiter who adopts a façade to please customers and then to be tipped. The waiter adopts a role, and mask. Sartre describes this as acting in "bad faith" or engaging in self-deception by deceiving others. Sartre distinguishes between authenticity (the waiter who does not play act) and bad faith.

But Erving Goffman's (1990) dramaturgical model of social interaction would say that so-called "authenticity" is itself simply an example of expertise in "managing impressions". In medical education we call this the exercise of "professionalism". For Goffman, there is no dividing line between good and bad faith, rather there are polished and clumsy, or artful, and pedestrian, ways of managing impressions or presenting a "self", both "frontstage" (public) and "backstage" (private). Such a view, however, hollows out any ethical dimension to interactions and raises the question of who writes the scripts and to what ends? For Rancière (2013), those in whom power is invested clearly write the scripts of conventions of social exchange, so that an aesthetic of the multitude is displaced by a minority aesthetic of the élite. Here, sovereign power rules.

Again, medical students must learn how to manage feelings and present an appropriate professional front or demeanour in often intensive and pressing circumstances. Emotional labour, from the beginning of their education, is channelled and formed according to "professional" expectations. Such capital is no longer owned by the students but becomes the property of the institutions of the medical school and the clinic (the medical hierarchy). It is redistributed according to historically determined patterns of expected professional behaviour. Such emotional or affective capital is intimately linked with sense-based dispositions and actions (perceiving, feeling, making value judgements, developing tastes) that Rancière (2006b, 2010) calls "the fabric of the sensible". Such a personal perceptual scheme, and associated social code of manners, is subject to a power structure, or is "policed". Such policing is based on time-honoured and loose traditions of apprenticeship or work-based learning – often diffuse and ill-conceived, lacking even basic frames such as briefing and de-briefing.

Breaches of professionalism are serious in the socialisation of trainee doctors, so much so that medical students themselves can come to police the behaviour of their seniors if they spot such breaches. These may be reported back to core medical school faculty who in turn can police the pedagogical behaviour of clinical teachers. These interactions then form a fabric of the sensible through highly structured and coded patterns of distribution of emotional capital, as acts of governance and counter-resistance (Gill et al. 2015; Monrouxe et al. 2014; Shaw et al. 2018). Such interactions involve both politics and aesthetics – or power and sensibility. And centrally, as in breaches of professionalism, ethics enters the scene.

Rancière (2013: ix) describes aesthetics broadly as "ways of perceiving and being affected", where again boundaries or transgressions are "policed". Tyson Lewis (2012: 1) describes the cultural "system of divisions and boundaries ... that define what is visible and audible within a particular aesthetico-political regime". Lewis would include here all the senses, or their interactions, to form a fabric of the senses as: "an organizational system of co-ordinates that establishes a distribution of the sensible" (ibid.: 3). The novelist China Miéville (2018) describes the education of sensibility as "reconfigurations of experience" in accordance with the habits of a dominant social group.

In *The Politics of Aesthetics*, Rancière (2006b: 50) notes that the relations between power and sensibility are not grounded in some transcendental abstract principles (as Kant insisted), but are immanent, fluid, and subject to historical conditions: "The visibility of a form of expression as an artistic form depends on a historically constituted regime of perception and intelligibility". Medical students (who have signed up for a vocational programme) effectively work for, or are employees of, medical schools in conjunction with university hospitals and primary care facilities (the latter in the UK served by regional postgraduate Deaneries that organise work placements and continuing professional development including qualifying as a doctor and being registered as such, and movement into specialties or into primary care). They are educated in time to adapt largely to hospital performance spaces: clinics, operating theatres, admissions units, intensive or critical care units, Accident and Emergency units, both generalist and specialty-based wards, and inter-disciplinary team meetings.

They know relatively little of how the patients they meet also circulate through a medical system as a complex web of associations: primarily as electronic medical records; as blood or tissue samples, through pathology laboratory spaces; as discharged patients through physiotherapy or support services; as admissions through ambulance and paramedic services; or as patients discharged into the community and cared for by social services, community services, and formal and informal carers. More, they know little of object-oriented ontologies that treat these circulating objects (such as human tissue or patients' notes) without objectifying them, while having equal ontological status within a system of practice (Harman 2018; Mol 2002). They come to know a little about social care, palliative care, and nursing homes, and more about family or general practice. Their physical, intellectual, and emotional labour is then focused clinically.

As they progress in their careers to medicine or surgery, and then to specialties (including general practice), what Tyson Lewis (2012) calls "acclimation pedagogy" – focused on work-based learning – intensifies. This is a pedagogy that does not primarily open an inquiring mind and teach critical thinking. Rather, it is one that narrows down learning to specifics that are tightly policed or subject to a strong ethical and professional frame, following a pattern of induction and sociali-sation. It is a classic case of the machinations of a professional apparatus of what Louis Althusser called "ideological interpellation" – the invisible assimilation of dominant cultural values in the absence of an explicit persuasive act. Ideologies are soaked up through a kind of osmosis. This is how medical students not only learn medicine, but how to adopt the identity of a doctor or a surgeon within classi-cally hierarchical structures. Performance spaces (Bleakley 2016) – such as operat-ing theatres, morgues, laboratories, wards, critical care units, dermatology clinics, maternity units, lecture theatres, and so forth – cultivate ways of emoting and being that are tightly controlled by conventions and traditions, where emotional capital is held by an authority and a fabric of sensibility is formed so that you sense according to how you should and not necessarily how you wish, as a circulation of tradition. Ironically, the major policing device of biomedical science as this affects clinical practice – the authoritative and sovereign power that is "evidence-based practice" – is consistently resisted by the facilitative and capillary power of "practice-based evidence". The latter is, colloquially, "the way we do things around here" as local habits or customs (Gabbay and le May 2016; Wieringa and Greenhalgh 2015).

Modes of perception and regimes of emotion tailored historically for special-ties are performance scripts demanding close reading leading to an identity con-struction. But, of course, change and progress must happen, and this is not just knowledge- or technique-based. Styles and approaches change too, and for such innovations to happen the fabric of the sensible must be rented and sensibility capital must be re-distributed. Forms of counter-resistance seed such innovations. Medical culture shifts from the default position of a "will-to-stability" to seek "pos-sibility knowledge" ("spearheads") through forms of political resistance, a model I emphasise throughout this book (Engeström 2018).

This can happen in a large-scale shift of values, such as democratisation of medicine through patient-centredness and inter-professional practices – both engi-neered and promoted by medical education. Lewis (2012) describes how "the aes-thetic principle of democracy" by its very nature breaches acclimation pedagogy. Here – as Michael Hardt and Antonio Negri (2000, 2006, 2009, 2017) describe – "Empire" morphs into "Multitude" then "Common Wealth" and finally "Assem-bly" as historical processes of democratisation intensify and are refined. (If Jacques Rancière's work is central to understanding how politics and aesthetics interplay in life, so Hardt and Negri advertise how politics and ethics intertwine). This follows Hegel's evolution of Spirit or Mind through dialectic, as the passage from individu-alism to collectivism (as shared values and co-existent mindset), and Marx's evolu-tion of social equity as common ownership of the means of production of goods, services, ideas, and emotional capital. This is echoed in collaborative, democratic pedagogical practices such as small group learning with student-led components.

Aesthetic labour

Aesthetic labour, introduced earlier, is commonly associated with service industries and the world of fashion, where organisations come to control the self-presentation of their workers in line with top-down dictated practices. This includes how one dresses, speaks, interacts with customers and fellow workers, and so forth. Grugulis, Warhurst and Keep (2004) argue "there is an increasing tendency for organisations to manage the way their employees feel and look as well as the way they behave", so that work is emotional and aesthetic as well as (or instead of) productive (see Hochschild 1983; Macdonald and Sirianni 1996; Warhurst and Nickson 2020).

The medical humanities provide frameworks for better understanding and appreciating differing kinds of work in medicine such as "affective labour" and "aesthetic labour". Affective labour involves both chronic-accumulative and acute exercise of affect or feelings, typical of medical work. Aesthetic labour involves both chronic-accumulative and acute exercise of the senses, in ways that engage form and beauty – again, typical of medical work.

Ten kinds of aesthetic work

The sum of the intersections between medicine, medical education, politics, and aesthetics can then be framed as the work of the medical humanities (Bleakley 2015, 2019; Bleakley, Marshall and Brömer 2006). Aesthetics in medicine – and not "aesthetic medicine and surgery" as corrective, or as embellishment and enhancement – is a minefield and rarely discussed in medical education. With some notable exceptions (Bleakley 2017; Macneill 2014; O'Neill 2015), even the field of the medical humanities resists in-depth discussion of aesthetics. While medical ethics – the issue of moral principles guiding practices and choices – is established in medical education, aesthetics is not yet afforded a similar status. Yet, as the opening account of this chapter advertises, ethics and aesthetics are inextricably mixed, where what is valued is a mix of a job done thoughtfully and sensitively (ethics), and well – or work of quality (aesthetics). Aesthetics has lost its tether and become inflated where it is seen to refer to high art rather than the *quality* and *form* of activity based in close noticing or cultivation of the senses, as sensibility (Bleakley 2020b).

As noted previously, the root of the word "aesthetic" is the ancient Greek *aisthesis* – "sense impression", meaning experience gained directly through perception and sensation without cognitive interpretation or interference. As a formal modern study, aesthetics began with the German philosopher Alexander Baumgarten's particular use of the word in 1735 to describe refined responses to high art or the appreciation of beauty. But the approach described here goes beyond the root meaning of the word, that, as noted, is to engage the senses fully – precisely what doctors do in conducting a physical or mental examination and making a diagnosis for example. While aesthetics is now used to describe qualities and form, this can range across a spectrum of emotional and sensory responses to embrace disgust as well as pleasure.

Thus, in medical education, the aesthetic realm can include dealing with disgust in clinical encounters with wounds, disease, and death, as well as the sensory pleasures of watching someone return to health. Aesthetics describes the education of the senses to make finer discriminatory clinical judgements, for example through auscultation, percussion, and palpation, as well as close observation and smell (ibid.).

In medical education, aesthetics is a lost or unknown territory, now controlled by instrumental concerns. This is understandable where scientific medicine has displaced interest in form and appearance for dominance of function. Appreciation of form has then been an-aesthetised or dulled rather than aestheticised. Good anatomy and applied science teachers cannot have lost their wonder at the display of the natural world, yet this aesthetic response will usually be lost where explanation precedes appreciation, rather than the other way around. I would recommend that those teachers embed themselves in the work of the biologist Adolf Portmann (for example 1967) – who argues for appreciation preceding explanation in biology – to restore a sense of wonder to their interests. Typically, Portmann resists the reduction of form to function, such as the territorial explanation for birdsong. Much of birdsong, suggests Portmann, is for the sake of it – expression of beauty rather than fence-building, that smells too much in any case of human capitalist interests projected onto the animal world.

Below, I consider ten kinds of aesthetic that can, and should, engage medical education. Each of these is entangled with politics or power, and ethics or value choices.

1   Appreciation of science
    The science informing medical practice is explanatory, but science should not be reduced to function alone (my mantra should now be familiar to readers). Science should be appreciated for its beauty, and natural wonders for their expression. Natural science precedes and embraces experimental and laboratory science. There are however ethical issues to consider – pathologised tissue may look beautiful under the microscope, but this tissue is from a person's body and being, and that person may be suffering. Electron microscopy images are generally stunning, but this is not how we normally see the world.
2   Modification of the senses
    As discussed in other chapters, medical students undergo a radical re-orientation of the senses, dictated by the authority of medical education, to which they must willingly submit to eventually attain a medical identity. A whole slice of sensibility concerned with disgust and revulsion must be re-educated to accept what will be a daily part of an assault on the senses – illness, wounding, bodily harm, and death. The primary aesthetic education is then an an-aesthetising or dulling of the ordinary. In parallel, however, is an education of an extraordinary sensibility and sensitivity to suffering and hurt – and a celebration of return to health through treatment – as these are presented in symptom patterns for close diagnostic noticing.

3 Democracy

Engaging democracy is an art and evolving. Democracy is a project, such that it is often described as a "democracy-to-come". Globally, for example, state democracies are in the minority. In the face of historical traditions of hierarchies within medicine broadly and within specialties, particularly in surgery, medical students are encouraged to develop democracies of patient-centredness and inter-professionalism. But these ideal end states are far from being achieved, again as democracies-to-come. However, there is a strong evidence base that flattening hierarchies in healthcare creates conditions for improved patient outcomes, safety, and worker satisfaction (Green et al. 2017). The blunt tactics of authority-led or arrogant behaviour are devoid of art where the latter demands high tolerance of ambiguity, absent in the former. Democratic debate, collaboration, and work of consensus require artful reflection and adjustment.

4 Clinical judgement

Students and junior doctors develop formed diagnostic capabilities as they progress. Balancing normative scientific evidence (guidelines) and personal judgement about the individual patient is an art – the forming of "mindlines" (Gabbay and le May 2016) as discussed earlier, or clinical judgement based largely on experience and local tradition rather than strictly on evidence-based clinical guidelines. Again, this is practice-based evidence rather than evidence-based practice.

5 Cultural Style

Style is a cohesive set of qualities, such as the Minimalism that characterises the clinical space, and the reporting styles of doctors – brief and to the point.

6 Personal style or taste

This is what characterises the individual clinician, to include innovations, adaptability, and improvisation. Value judgements are appropriate to context (ethical and sensitive). While taste is often reduced to relativism (personal taste), there is a common factor. Taste is essential to medical diagnostics, where a blunt or dulled range of senses makes for a poor diagnostic radar.

7 Beauty

Words such as "form", "elegance", and "beauty" do not readily roll off the tongues of hard-pressed and/or hard-bitten doctors. "Beauty" has its root in the Latin *bellus*, meaning "fine" or "refined". Medicine is a fine art and a refined application of science and humanities. Nobody wants a medicine that is clumsy, dull, or ugly.

8 Cognition and creativity

Medical education above all aims to engage a creative imagination that moves beyond conservatism and a will-to-stability in learning to nurture innovation and possibility knowledge.

9 Resistance

Acts of resistance to perceived injustices, sleights, or abuse of power and authority (dissensus rather than consensus) can power creative change or modification or turn the ordinary into the extraordinary. The arts and humanities are identified by their powers of dissensus, to make us "think otherwise". Individuals may cultivate sophisticated forms of resistance to perceived injustices and authorities such as "sly civility", a mocking of authority disguised as conformity.

10 Appearance

Self-presentation affords a trustworthy impression for patients and colleagues. Doctors want to appear professional and confident, but not arrogant. Management of impressions is an art and medicine can be readily understood as theatre, with tight scripts and specific roles. In fact, soap opera representations of medicine ("medi-soaps") are one way that the public can be informed about medical culture while retaining value as entertainment. Once a vocation but now a job, doctors manage appearances in a broader variety of ways than in previous generations, and this is inflected particularly by the disappearance of major props such as the white coat and stethoscope. We need, however, to go beyond surface appearance to authenticity, or Heiddegerian Being, as the micro-political acts of what Michel Foucault (2005) calls "aesthetic (and ethical) self-forming". Just as a practice is formed aesthetically, or has contour, grace, and beauty, so an identity is formed – not just informed "doctor", or "surgeon", but also "professional" and "trustworthy person".

Sensibility is first cultural capital before it is personal taste, open to forms of resistance (see Figures 7.1–7.3). When a medical student unlearns (represses) a response of disgust to bodily fluids for example, senior members of the profession

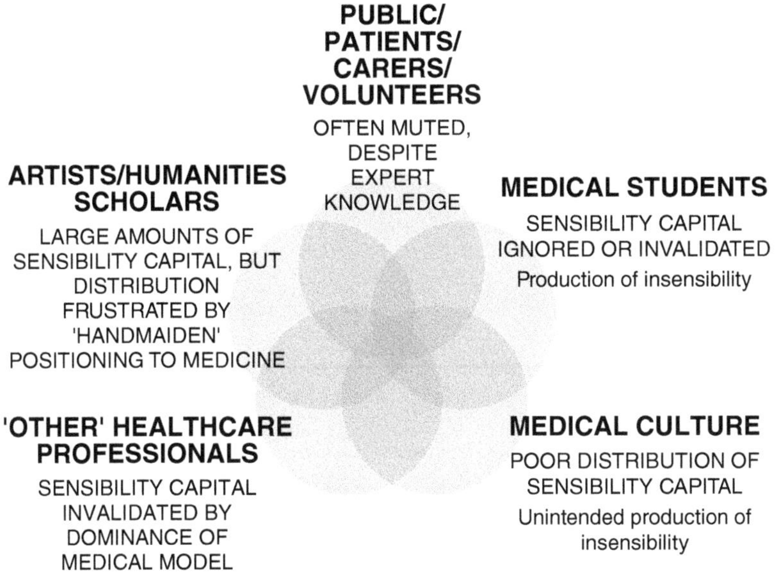

**PUBLIC/
PATIENTS/
CARERS/
VOLUNTEERS**
OFTEN MUTED,
DESPITE
EXPERT
KNOWLEDGE

**ARTISTS/HUMANITIES
SCHOLARS**
LARGE AMOUNTS OF
SENSIBILITY CAPITAL, BUT
DISTRIBUTION
FRUSTRATED BY
'HANDMAIDEN'
POSITIONING TO MEDICINE

MEDICAL STUDENTS
SENSIBILITY CAPITAL
IGNORED OR INVALIDATED
Production of insensibility

**'OTHER' HEALTHCARE
PROFESSIONALS**
SENSIBILITY CAPITAL
INVALIDATED BY
DOMINANCE OF
MEDICAL MODEL

MEDICAL CULTURE
POOR DISTRIBUTION OF
SENSIBILITY CAPITAL
Unintended production of
insensibility

FIGURE 7.1 Mapping the distribution of sensibility capital

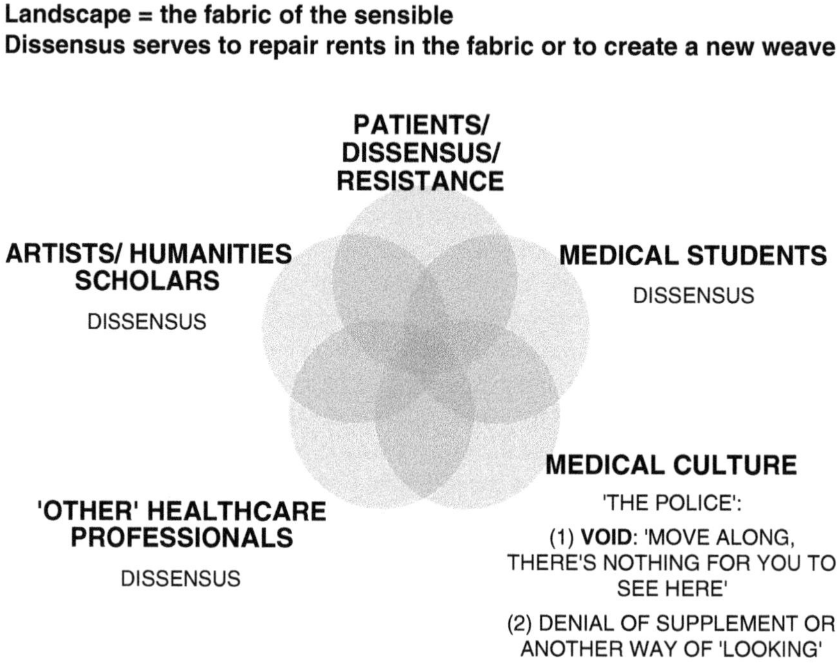

Landscape = the fabric of the sensible
Dissensus serves to repair rents in the fabric or to create a new weave

PATIENTS/
DISSENSUS/
RESISTANCE

ARTISTS/ HUMANITIES
SCHOLARS

DISSENSUS

MEDICAL STUDENTS

DISSENSUS

MEDICAL CULTURE

'THE POLICE':

(1) **VOID**: 'MOVE ALONG,
THERE'S NOTHING FOR YOU TO
SEE HERE'

(2) DENIAL OF SUPPLEMENT OR
ANOTHER WAY OF 'LOOKING'

'OTHER' HEALTHCARE
PROFESSIONALS

DISSENSUS

FIGURE 7.2   Forms of dissensus or resistance

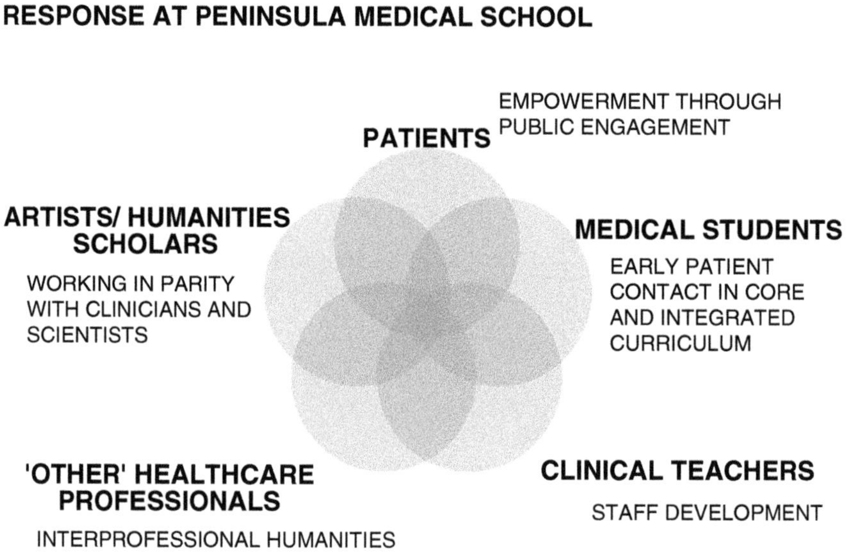

RESPONSE AT PENINSULA MEDICAL SCHOOL

EMPOWERMENT THROUGH
PATIENTS PUBLIC ENGAGEMENT

ARTISTS/ HUMANITIES
SCHOLARS

WORKING IN PARITY
WITH CLINICIANS AND
SCIENTISTS

MEDICAL STUDENTS

EARLY PATIENT
CONTACT IN CORE
AND INTEGRATED
CURRICULUM

'OTHER' HEALTHCARE
PROFESSIONALS

INTERPROFESSIONAL HUMANITIES

CLINICAL TEACHERS

STAFF DEVELOPMENT

FIGURE 7.3   Specific institutional resistance to traditional forms of distribution of
sensibility capital

– as teachers, mentors, and role models – effectively drain off the emotional capital involved to retain this, as in a classic psychoanalytic transference process. In return, seniors are allowed to express emotion openly, sometimes as fiery criticism, sarcastic comment, or jibe. Again, the distribution of emotional capital is frustrated where it is retained in the lore of the elders and conservation of bad habits, and the emotional responses of neophytes are seen as illegitimate or do not constitute legitimate capital. While symptoms of unprofessionalism include objectification of patients, overt cynicism, and historical ritual humiliation of juniors such as "pimping", they also embrace the other end of the spectrum as lack of emotional insulation and over-involvement with patients. In other words, both ends of the spectrum (under- and over-involvement) demonstrate insensibility. Figure 7.1 summarises various faces of the distribution of sensibility capital in medicine and medical education according to historically determined or traditional power structures. Figure 7.2 illustrates how patterns of resistance can emerge, while Figure 7.3 relates such patterns to a specific institution.

Acclimation pedagogies

Returning to the (mal)distribution of sensibility capital, introduced in the first part of this chapter, acclimation (American usage) or acclimatisation (British usage) is the process and result of becoming accustomed to a new climate or to new conditions. Lewis (2012) describes "acclimation pedagogy" as the formalised learning of an identity or new way of being on the terms of an externally imposed authority.

In China Miéville's (2009) novel *The City & The City*, two cities sit side-by-side with differing cultures and languages. At points they overlap ("crosshatching" and living "grosstopically"). Growing up in either city requires learning how to "unsee" members of the other city and its infrastructure. This is an acclimation (or acclimatising) process. Prospective travellers to either city undergo intensive acclimation pedagogy before they are given visas. Should a citizen of either city consciously or inadvertently "see" the other city and its inhabitants, this is called "breaching" and the person is immediately arrested by the Breach police and given re-education in perception, in how to sense appropriately and selectively. Persistent breaching leads to more severe punishment. The novel offers a metaphor for the shaping of the senses by culture and history. Aesthetics, as the manipulation of the sensible fabric of the world and responses to qualities, are historically and culturally inflected. There is a mild echo here too of senior doctors embedded in specialties who are discouraged from trespassing on the territories of others' specialties.

There is nothing necessarily sinister about this – we are subject to learning new sensibility practices through external authority all the time. Lockdown and social distancing in a climate of emergency are recent global examples. Vigilance in the face of "terrorist threat" is another. All professional socialisations, or regimes of formal rule-bound activity such as sports, require acclimation. The point is to be reflexive about patterns and possibilities. Where does an acclimation pedagogy become an oppressive socialisation, frustrate innovation, or slowly erode patience and resilience through micro-aggressions?

Socialisation into medicine requires divesting oneself of key lay emotional capital (ways of being) and intellectual capital (ways of thinking and problem solving) to engage with the professional culture that is oriented to emotional insulation (potentially numbing empathy) and practical action (potentially numbing conceptual acuity). It is a process of unlearning one set of habits to learn a new set. An important work of political resistance occurs as medical students retain personal signifiers in the face of medical socialisation. Millenials and Generation Z medical students and junior doctors may come to constitute the force of resistance that radically changes the nature of medical education post-coronavirus pandemic. The inevitable social change post-pandemic must surely alert medical education to the central importance of health eco-literacy and radical "upstream" medicine where the climate emergency can be seen as a pandemic in slow motion (Bleakley 2021).

Emotional (or affective) capital, produced from emotional labour (Brook 2013; Hochschild 1983), is extremely important in medical education. Such capital is central to how communication is exercised, and communication is key to patient care and safety. As noted previously, in recent years we have accrued research evidence that most medical errors or iatrogenic mistakes are products of poor communication not between doctors and patients, but between doctors and other healthcare professionals in "liquid" clinical team settings – fast paced clinical encounters with little room for error. This is particularly acute in surgical settings, both within and across teams (Bleakley 2013).

Such a draining-off of affective capital has consequences – medical students feel dried out and dehumanised, just as patients might. Here, medicine has developed professional codes and engineered climates of democracy: patient-centredness and inter-professional teamwork. Students expect seniors to model professional behaviour as sensitivity to patients. In most cases, seniors do this well. When they do not, students can and do organise modes of political resistance to recover emotional capital that has been lodged in the apex of the hierarchy. For example, contra acclimation, students do not necessarily "unsee" professional lapses by seniors and are ready to report perceived unprofessional behaviour, and in the worse cases to whistle-blow.

Intellectual knowing and practical doing are held together by affective glue, by feelings and sentiments. The easiest way to test this is to look at symptoms of breakdown or burnout (Peterkin and Bleakley 2017). Knowledge and practices are valued for their qualities, and it is the value complex that holds a practice together. If the practice is devalued, then the practitioner loses interest. Around any set of practices, a web of values forms that holds the practices and these are represented in medical aphorisms ("patient-centredness", "do no harm", "treat the person not the disease") (Levine and Bleakley 2012). This affective glue represents a set of interests that are "formed" or "shaped", and that form an identity in turn. This shaping gives qualities to a practice such as elegance, sensitivity, assuredness, and so forth. The quality of a practice is its aesthetic dimension, readily known by how it engages the senses. Where senses are tuned, there is vibrancy and readiness, or an aesthetic presence. Where senses are dulled, there is a bluntness or dullness, and practice is an-aesthetised.

Any set of practices underpinned by knowledge and values, such as medicine and medical pedagogies, can be seen to form a fabric, a connectedness. These fabrics are also known by their locations: the hospital ward, clinic, and operating theatre; the primary care clinic; the hospice. Often this fabric of the sensible is heavily specialised, such as a paediatric audiology clinic with video playback facilities for observing how parents interact with a deaf child. The fabric embraces practitioners and family members engaging in affect-laden work around a child to seek possibility knowledge as parents learn new ways of communicating and the child gains confidence.

Grit and pearls

As we have seen from previous chapters, for some, the medical humanities (or health humanities) have a beguiling charm as a distraction from the blood and guts of clinical medicine, bringing some sophistication also to the blunt instrumentalism of applied biomedical science. Patients are portraits and stories, their symptoms poetry, while everyday clinical procedures afford notable drama. These are the pearls of the medical humanities beyond the grit of everyday medical work that does not engage a creative imagination or pursuit of possibility knowledge. But this is to idealise the medical humanities and we must stand this view on its head. There is common grit that makes these pearls. This is the medical humanities as collective workhorse – bringing the fullness of humanity to medicine in the form of democracy at work within medical education. Central to this is (often bruising) politics – the machinations of power. Medical humanities interventions produce tangible productive effects (Mangione et al. 2018) because blood, sweat and tears are involved. Often caricatured as play, the medical humanities demand work – they are a specialised form of labour. As labour, they offer capital to the medical humanities employers, medicine itself. Historically, we have seen that medicine has claimed the labour of the medical humanities for itself, or has poached the capital of the medical humanities, where it sees the medical humanities as pleasant diversion or supportive act. The medical humanities in medical education have always had to work hard, swimming against the tide, proving their worth, bearing the weight of scepticism, and so forth.

Politics is often cast as the intrusive shadow of medicine and medical pedagogy that can turn artistry into sinister Machiavellian power plays. This is akin to what William Blake called the "infernal machine" or Chiaro Oscuro, the "hellish" brown shadows beloved by Venetian and Flemish painters that Blake saw as a mean-spirited treacle coating, denying potential light and illumination. Politics in medicine – most immediately in policy and healthcare management – need not be sticky brown shadows. Indeed, it is time to bring politics out of the shadows and celebrate power in medicine and medical pedagogies as potentially liberatory; and, certainly, as terrains for artful resistance to heavy-handed and unimaginative pedagogies, particularly in curriculum development, where medical education has shown a strange resistance to contemporary innovations.

More, where it situates such innovative thinking in the field of medical humanities, this constitutes a "thinking-politics-with-curriculum-in-mind" as a poetic device. To repeat my mantra – now, hopefully, plainly evident to readers – here politics and aesthetics meet such that power is not conceived as blunt, material, and instrumental (acting as an an-aesthetic) but rather as an aesthetic gesture that shapes democratic habits as things of beauty and elegance, awakening the senses. The curriculum is then not dull and dulling, but sharp, pointed, challenging and enervating. It is an approach to curriculum that should enlighten and needle at the same time. Such a curriculum literally makes sense, raising levels of sensibility to create medical students who are alive to what patients want, or have their antennae up.

The medical/health humanities have been shown to educate the sensibilities and sensitivities of medical students as a platform for improving clinical diagnostic capabilities and shaping doctors who listen to their patients and respond caringly. But this work, to which I have contributed (for example Bleakley 2015, 2019, 2020a), is limited by its previous refusal to engage with politics or power structures. Despite a global interest in incorporating medical humanities in medicine and surgery curricula there is a danger of producing dilettante pearl fishers rather than artisanal grit shifters, the former perhaps interested more in the delicate intricacies of narrative theory or obscure historical fact rather than the everyday incessant noises of power plays and resistances that characterise both the joys and tensions of clinical work. We must wrestle the medical humanities away from the medical gaze and away from para-ownership by medical culture serving to reduce the medical humanities, again, to handmaiden status. Another way of looking at this is, again, to encourage biomedically inspired medicine to up its game, to intensify and complexify in embracing a shift in values from the instrumental to a deeper register embracing the aesthetic, political and ethical.

In this chapter, I have placed emphasis on the values sphere of the political. Crudely, I want to encourage a shift in gaze of the medical humanities from art gallery to contemporary eco-factory, and of medical education generally from downstream hospitalism, or hospital-based work experience, to upstream primary care and "deep upstream" community care focused on the long-term implications of an ecological crisis as an exploitation of common wealth by cynical private interests. Again, such exploitation supports and deepens health inequities and inequalities. I have written about this extensively elsewhere (Bleakley 2021).

Hegel's Master: Slave formula says there is no master without the slave. In other words, the slave affords the master's *raison d'être*. This gives the slave a paradoxical power. Without customers there are no shopkeepers. Without the populus or multitude there are no politicians. Without patients there are no doctors. And without medical students there are no medical educators. Medical students have power because they provide the medium through which medical educators can continually transform and develop their pedagogies. Jacques Rancière's (1991) *The Ignorant Schoolmaster* posits a pedagogical thought experiment: what if the teacher knew the same as, or even less than, the pupils? This appears ridiculous in terms of specialist factual knowledge; but it is worth considering in terms of how facts are translated into clinical work where patient and colleague interactions are important.

How would teaching and learning progress if teaching were made redundant? The point is to bring our focus back to the resources that are provided by learners and the potential for adapting content-heavy curricula into "learning to learn" processes. "Teaching" then becomes "facilitation of learning". More radical approaches to such a pedagogy develop collaborative inquiry as the primary mode of learning (what we need to know and how we can best learn this in collective contexts), and criteria-based self and peer assessment as the most democratic ways of judging whether learning has taken place, and if expertise is being acquired. To traditionalists, none of this would make sense – it would be senseless. But this chapter, I hope, has demonstrated that sense is common, or beyond property. As such, sense capital can be distributed in ways that challenge historical hierarchies and patterns of ownership. In medical education, the revolution cannot come quickly enough.

8

UNDERSTANDING "PRESCRIPTION CULTURE" THROUGH LITERATURE

Metaphors as pills

This chapter presents an extended case study of how the medical humanities can "work" within a medicine and surgery undergraduate curriculum, taking on the collective role of mediator and translator between biomedical science and clinical practice. The work of translation, as we have seen, is one of increasing quality, intensity, and complexity of thinking and practice, where reductive instrumentalism in either biomedicine or clinical practice is challenged. In the process of translation, the productive metaphor count is increased, and metaphor innovation is enhanced.

Prescribing is an aspect of undergraduate medical education that is consistently reported as poorly taught or neglected in curricula (Ross and Maxwell 2012). Pharmacists are rarely brought in to teach medical students, while pharmacy students and medical students rarely work together collaboratively. Further, prescribing is commonly taught free from consideration of ethical problems such as considering potential addictions (Singh and Pushkin 2019) – highlighted recently by the opioid crisis, particularly in the USA (Bleakley 2021). The medical humanities can offer a way of "thinking otherwise" or looking "slant" (to draw on the poet Emily Dickinson's term) at a topic that could so readily be reduced to instrumental listings or functional information. Medical students will learn little about pharmaceutical treatments for mental health issues and will probably not be encouraged to match qualitative case study perceptions of the unique with population study metrics and generalised descriptions of drug effects and side effects. The general case rarely fully matches the individual case.

Pharmaceuticals are translational devices. In the case of the drugs discussed in this chapter, they are mood enhancers that promise "better living through

DOI: 10.4324/9781003383260-9

chemistry" – a euphemistic term for recreational drug use. The phrase was adapted from the pharma giant DuPont's advertising slogan in the 1930s "Better Things for Better Living Through Chemistry" and taken up – as "better living through chemistry" – in 1996 by the DJ Fatboy Slim (Norman Cook) as the title of his first (electronic dance) album. DuPont dropped their imaginative tagline in 1999 for the bland "the miracles of science".

Pharmaceuticals are perhaps better described as catalysts rather than translators, for they remain unchanged (while of course they are ingested and incorporated) while the person who ingests them changes, for better or worse. Such drugs are certainly active objects, extensions of the consciousness/bodily state of those who ingest them as well as extensions of the pharmaceutical company who produce them, thus acting as mobile capital within several economies (mind, body, culture, capitalism) including the aesthetic economy. Such drugs shape qualities, for better or worse. The origin of the English word "drug" is from the Middle Dutch *droge vate* ("dry vats") and the Old French *drogue*, referring to the contents of such vats, as "dry goods". If experience is the container, drugs are by turns welcome, unexpected, and unwelcome guests. Just as such "dry goods" are exchanged and trafficked in the outer markets, so they circulate across the synapses of the brain and display in the psyche, proving to be better or worse investments.

Prescription culture amongst harassed, overworked doctors is a topic for concern. For example, General Practitioners (GPs) in the UK are "giving antidepressants to children against guidelines" as one newspaper headline has it (Campbell 2022). Children as young as 11 are regularly being prescribed antidepressants rather than talking therapies. GPs say this is because of the backlog in getting children seen by child and adolescent psychiatry services. Up to 30,000 children may now be regularly taking antidepressants for anxiety and depression in the UK (ibid.). Meanwhile, Matt Richtel (2022), in the *New York Times,* describes "A generation of guinea pigs" where "depressed adolescents are being prescribed multiple psychiatric drugs". The article begins:

One morning in the fall of 2017, Renae Smith, a high school freshman on Long Island in New York, could not get out of bed, overwhelmed at the prospect of going to school. In the following days, her anxiety mounted into despair.

Renae described her pain, creating a striking metaphor: "I cried, screamed and begged the universe or whatever godly power to take away the pain of a thousand men that was trapped inside my head".

A psychoanalyst – thinking of Freud's view of neurosis as the return of the repressed – might have made a good deal of the analogy of a thousand trapped men, but here, let's just stick with what happened next in Renae's tale. After a visit to the local physician, Renae was transferred to a specialist in mental health, a psychiatrist, who prescribed Prozac (Fluoxetin), a notorious anti-depressant and cultural icon after Elizabeth Wurtzel's 1994 memoir *Prozac Nation* that spawned a film of the same name. Infamously, Wurtzel's personal-confessional account attracted caustic reviews for its self-indulgence and blatant narcissism. We cannot credit Wurtzel with inventing a genre of personal-confessional literature in which a drug attains the status of co-star with the author (this may go back to Thomas de Quincey's 1821 *Confessions of an English Opium-Eater*), but Wurtzel must gain credit for showing how anti-depressant and anti-anxiety pharmaceuticals became lifestyle choices for many rather than, primarily, medical interventions. Patients recovered their power in the doctor-patient encounter through a cultural effect. Pharmaceuticals of certain kinds could be understood, ingested, appreciated, and discussed critically without the shadow of patient "compliance" colouring the conversation. Patients want choice.

For Renae Smith, however, there seemed to be no choice as she became caught in a spiral of meek compliance. Her first prescription initiated a "medication cascade". By 2001, the year of her graduation from High School, Smith was taking seven prescribed drugs. Along with anti-depressant and anti-anxiety medication she was taking a drug to "stabilize mood" developed initially to control epileptic seizures and migraines (Smith suffered from neither of these conditions); and a drug to "dull the side-effects" of her five primary pharmaceuticals. Smith had joined many other young persons, mainly women, who are being prescribed multiple medications for what many may think is a typical feature of adolescence: mood swings, deep introspection, and psychological/emotional uncertainty, with periods of dip in affect (as opposed to debilitating clinical depression). Renae Smith is then part of an uncontrolled experiment in manipulation of the moods of young people through multiple chemical interventions at a time when compliance is also being severely challenged as citizens literally take ingestion of mood-defining pharmaceuticals into their own hands. We live in times of intense medical and recreational drug use. Doctors and medical students have joined the party. A 2008 literature review of illicit drug use amongst medical students in Brazil concluded: "The prevalence of licit and illicit drug use among medical students is high, even though they understand the injuries it may cause" (Candido et al. 2008: 462).

Renae Smith's symptoms, typically, scooped up attention deficit hyperactivity disorder (ADHD) to add to mood "disorders". As we shall see later, ADHD has become a mini epidemic amongst younger persons, raising the spectre that it is a condition partly invented by the major pharmaceutical companies, in league with some psychiatrists, to sell more drugs. Smith's prescriptions now covered the spectrum of ADHD, depression, anxiety, mood disorders including bipolar disorder, psychotropics used to treat schizophrenia, and seizure and migraine medication. Of course, dosage is key here, and most of the drugs would be prescribed in low dosage. But their potential interactions are largely uncharted. Smith was not so much being treated as being transformed into something that she did not envisage when first given Prozac. Increasingly, she suffered from suicidal ideation – but it was now impossible to know whether this was a product of her ragbag of medications or a genuine call of the soul beyond "better living through chemistry".

Smith, concerned at the escalating size of her pharmaceutical cavalry, sought out a "talking therapy" psychiatrist who weaned her off the meds, just as she received a diagnosis of a developing thyroid cancer. The uncertainty of her condition, while thrown into a parallel and unscheduled treatment regime including surgery for the cancer, served to reinforce her desire to wean herself off the medley of meds. At the time of volunteering to be the subject of *The New York Times* article from which I am quoting, she had reduced her intake to two daily drugs – one for ADHD and one for depression. She also took an anti-anxiety med if symptoms flared – around once a week in her own account. Her everyday concerns were now focused on gaining a place at a local Community College to study for a degree in environmental and wildlife sciences. This seems significant, as a turn to outer, ecological concerns began to replace some years of ego-logical self-absorption.

This single case is typical – there is a large literature on the booming caseload of mental health issues worldwide. UK General (Family) Practitioners in more deprived areas find that their caseload is now around 40% of psychosomatic/mental health presentations. Yet, undergraduate medical education provides woeful preparation for this, where it excludes attention to educating for psychotherapeutic capabilities (Bleakley 2021). Further, as David Haslam (2020: 26) notes, "In countries around the world, research is being undertaken into the concept of low-value care, typically defined as an intervention where evidence suggests it confers little or no benefit on patients". In fact, this may bleed into iatrogenesis – where the medical intervention itself produces symptoms that need to be treated (such as debilitating side effects of drugs). Certainly, following the grain of my account that opens this chapter, while it is the case that many people suffer from debilitating symptoms of depression and anxiety and benefit from pharmaceutical therapies, as many patients again may benefit from purely psychotherapeutic interventions and community support.

Caught in a classic double-bind, high-income countries in particular – bent on "high achievement" – produce the very conditions that can stifle such achievement: stress and concomitant permeating anxiety and inevitable depression. "Inevitable" because we raise the bar too high for success and many people simply cannot reach that bar and feel depressed because of it. Or, because of structural factors, access is denied to such high bar "success", where inability to achieve such unrealistic standards may be felt as failure. A medical consequence of this double bind is, again, high rates of prescription by GPs of anti-anxiety and anti-depression drugs. In fact, there is an epidemic of such mental health conditions (demand) paired with an insatiable supply chain formed out of Big Pharma's desire for profits and (mainly) general or family practitioners' succumbing to short-term, instrumental fixes for conditions that have structural causes and demand more complex psychosocial treatments.

Killing two birds with one drug, selective serotonin reuptake inhibitors (SSRIs) treat both anxiety and depression. The formal naming of these SSRI drugs is an interesting object of study, and, paradoxically, advertising a condition to be treated in itself – that of bottom-line instrumentalism, stripped of quality or aesthetic. For example, the anti-anxiety sedative group of benzodiazepines derive this generic name from their chemical structure of a benzene ring and a diazepine ring. Where it may tickle the fancy of biochemists, this dull, formal bottom-line technical descriptor will neither inform lay patients nor excite poets. Better, poetically, that we give some texture to the topic by talking in terms of popular, or "street", names that act as metaphors, such as "uppers", "downers", "chill pills", and "tranks". "Benzodiazepines" as a biochemical descriptor doesn't capture the fact that these drugs are "tranquilisers" (tranks), conjuring images of tranquillity or quietude against a symptom background of racing anxiety. They are indeed "chill pills".

Medical students and doctors draw on regularly updated pharmaceutical formularies (in digital and print forms) for information about the drugs they prescribe for their patients, across somatic, psychosomatic, and psychological conditions. In the UK, this is the *British National Formulary* (BNF) a biannual joint publication of the British Medical Association and the Royal Pharmaceutical Society (bnf.nice.org.uk/). Such formularies are bottom-line technical or instrumental accounts, akin to engineering manuals or recipes. They contain quantitative data rather than descriptive qualitative data – for example, they are devoid of illustrative (and counter-illustrative) individual patient cases. For this reason, they present a readymade case study for the value of the medical humanities, where an aesthetic, political, or ethical values dimension can be brought to bear on a medical topic, raising its metaphor count, intensity, and quality.

To give an illustrative example, let us return to anti-anxiety drugs such as the benzodiazepines. An example is Alprazolam. You can look this up on your mobile phone by Googling "BNF" and then "Alprazolam". You will find that this drug is prescribed for "short-term use in anxiety". This is a linguistic conundrum, even a contradiction. Doesn't the contraction "short-term" immediately conjure up "anxiety" – connoting sudden cut-off rather than longer-term treatment? "Brief" therapies such as cognitive-behavioural therapy (CBT) conjure up a similar promise of short-termism rather than continued care, surely an echo of our short-attention-span culture? When Freud and Breuer shaped psychoanalysis, it became clear that this was less a short-term solution for neuroses (the analysis completed when the transference was resolved), but rather an educational life-course. Only the rich could afford this once- or twice-a-week therapeutic journey. This is why Alfred Adler (1870–1937), once a member of Freud's Vienna Circle, democratised psychotherapy by inventing what we now call "social work" and volunteer community support.

Returning to Alprazolam, reading the drug leaflet we find contradictions: a "paradoxical effect" of Alprazolam is "increase in hostility and aggression" and "increased anxiety". Excuse me? "Increased anxiety" is a possible side-effect of a drug that is given to reduce anxiety? Alice in Wonderland stuff. More, "increased anxiety" is a "common" or "very common" side effect of the drug. We too have gone down a disorienting rabbit hole with Alprazolam, better known by its trade name of Xanax. We shall meet this "better living through chemistry" drug later in this chapter as a character in contemporary literature. Xanax is not available on the UK's NHS although it can be prescribed in private medicine – a quirk in the British health system. It is a commonly prescribed drug in the USA, with nearly 20 million prescriptions annually. More commonly prescribed anti-anxiety drugs (anxiolytics) include Diazepam, perhaps better known as Valium. Xanax is ten times stronger than Valium. Yet the BNF reports the same "paradoxical effects" for Valium as for Xanax. Street names for Xanax include "ladders" because one's mood can go up and down. The rungs can become well worn. "Snakes" interact with the ladders as the illegal vendors of Xanax on the streets.

So, you can see already that a medical humanities lens can bring colour, depth, intensity, and social concern to the otherwise technical and instrumental biochemical outlook of the medics' and pharmacists' national formularies – books without any literary merit through expected content such as characters, metaphors, storylines, and poetic sensibility. Rather, formularies are dry, technical manuals. But need they be this way? Can we not increase the metaphor count, ratchet up portions of the text to give it some connection with life? This chapter will illustrate the value of the medical humanities by showing, first, that much can be learned about the relationship between the public, medicine, and prescription drugs from contemporary novelists; and second, that purely instrumental drug formularies (a staple of a doctor's armoury) can be given character through the inclusion of "living" case studies. In each case, medical students can benefit – from reading pertinent creative literature and from devising aspects of drug formularies (especially for drugs treating psychological conditions) that introduce case studies, so that the formulary is lifted from the purely instrumental to embrace other values perspectives.

Here is a conundrum. While most of the work of GPs is that of prescribing medicines, there is an assumption that patients are largely ignorant about what is prescribed. This may be the case for pharmaceuticals for bodily diseases, but it is not the case for drugs treating psychological or psychosomatic conditions. Here, the public body is well informed from popular culture, especially social media, including You Tube personal-confessional videos. There is also the recreational drug culture that presents the biggest paradox facing medicine, associated with street culture as an alternative clinic. While medicine sets out to prevent illness and to cure or manage illness, at the same time, the public body goes out of its way to get high or to seek relief from discomfort. It also goes out of its way to get ill, consuming bad food, engaging in dangerous activities, and shuttling sexually transmitted diseases. Medical students and doctors are part of that public body.

Medical students learn that one of their primary aids is a drug formulary – in the UK the BNF as noted above, updated every six months and including pharmaceuticals for both body and mind. Such formularies are the Ur-examples of functionalism and literalism in medicine. They are, again, purely informational. Not an ounce of aesthetic, ethical or political awareness seeps from between their covers. How then, might we re-vision and re-invigorate aspects of a drug formulary to remind medical students that both prescribed and "street"/recreational pharmaceuticals are imbibed by human beings with personalities and presences, where neither those humans nor the drugs they are taking should be treated mechanically? Recreational drugs are imbued with metaphor and personality – "daffy" (modafinil, a stimulant widely used by students – including medical students – for stamina during times of revision), "phennies" (barbiturates), "molly" (ecstasy), "special K" (ketamine), "acid" (LSD), "blow" (cocaine), and so forth. Drugs as mind-altering embodied metaphors – or metaphors as pills.

Again, the interactions between humans and pharmaceuticals cannot be reduced purely to chemistry (as they often are) but must be treated as ethical, aesthetic, political, and transcendental concerns. Chemistry itself is a reduction and must be returned to the contexts in which chemical reactions occur, and the consequences of such reactions. More, medical drugs always draw in economic concerns as there are costs involved. Sometimes this is critical, where a specific drug may be too costly to prescribe through normal health service channels. Further, drugs raise spiritual concerns. For example, recreational LSD, "magic mushrooms" (psylocybin) and other plant-based hallucinogens use has often been linked to religious epiphanies, while low dose psychedelics have been used in psychiatric and end of life care and continue to be researched for efficacy in treating chronic mental health conditions such as severe depression (Hunley undated). Pharmaceuticals are integral to our ways of being (ontologies) as translational media.

The first wave of the medical humanities – whose focus was the academic study of medicine and medical cultures (such as the history of medicine) – did not promise much in the way of translation into improving patient care. Rather, this wave gave a deeper understanding of the contexts in which medicine has developed and can be both appreciated and understood conceptually. A second wave of this approach to the medical humanities promises greater application. This current wave of interdisciplinary medical humanities engages critically with medicine as an ethical practice, and with ontologies of clinical practice, articulation of the historical conditions of possibility for the emergence of medical practices and approaches to health, development of a historical and cross-cultural appreciation of the body, and critical evaluation of the medicalisation of everyday behaviour. It is this last area of concern that is the focus of this chapter, and here the two streams of the historical-cultural medical humanities and the medical humanities in medical education engage in dialogue.

Prescription economies

The focus of the chapter is the development of a mental health "prescription culture" and its critical representation in contemporary novels and self-help books. By a mental health prescription culture, I mean a culture in which taking prescribed drugs for common psychosomatic symptoms such as anxiety and depression becomes a naturalised (and then unquestioned) part of the cultural fabric. In the northern hemisphere certainly, we live in a culture in which prescription drugs are discussed as separated out from the persons who are taking them, to become recognisable actors with distinct personalities. This is achieved through three main texts: medical pharmaceutical formularies, online confessional accounts such as *You Tube* videos, and contemporary literature. [There is, of course, a long tradition of the influence of, and the recounting of, drug use and abuse in literature – often called "addiction literature" – from Coleridge's 1816 *Kubla Khan* and Thomas De Quincey's 1821 *Confessions of an English Opium Eater* to the Beat Generation's William Burrough's 1953 *Junkie* and 1959 *The Naked Lunch*, and Alex Trocchi's 1960 *Cain's Book.*]

The development, administration, and evaluation of commonly taken anti-depressant and anti-anxiety drugs are part of the political regulation of sensibility, as discussed in the previous chapter. A critical view suggests that, largely driven by the profit motives of the pharmaceutical industry, psychological conditions continue to be medicalised and treated through a reductive neurological lens. Humans of course are readily essentialised to neurology, but as Alfred Adler insisted, the individual cannot be isolated from social contexts, historical influences, and cultural conditions.

As the fabric of the sensible (the aesthetic life) is patterned according to vested interests (the political and economic life) so an aesthetic of everyday life is shaped in which prescription culture has become a normal part of that fabric of the sensible. Indeed, although prescription drugs can be seen to be part of a cultural production of insensibility, they are advertised as producing precisely the opposite effect. They are promoted as relieving debilitating symptoms of depression and anxiety. This treatment of symptom misses the cause – that, for example, as noted above, living in a manic, sound-byte culture is bound to lower the threshold for what is considered a state of depression or one of anxiety. The bar for achievement remains impossibly high for many, while states of anomie and existential angst are part of the human condition, where "life is a bitch and then you die" (a street version of the American stand-up comedian George Carlin's line: "life is tough then you die"). Drugs of one kind or another can fill the gap, whether as psychological emollients or consciousness-raisers. Once ingested, the person becomes part of a web of sensible life that is partly controlled by the pharmaceutical industry and medical world. Your sensibility capital is to some extent dictated and remains in part under the ownership of the pharmaco-medical world.

As we saw in the previous chapter, Jacques Rancière (2013: ix–x) suggests, following Walter Benjamin, "forms of sensible experience" or "ways of perceiving and being affected" are subject to historical fluctuations. Those who exert power (authority figures or institutions, again such as medicine and the pharmaceutical industry) are the historical forces that shape or dictate legitimate forms of sensible experience. The fabric of the sensible, or how we shall perceive, is regulated. The major form of regulation is to produce insensibility in the general population as a form of policing, to dampen down the possibility of dissension or speaking out about ownership of the means of producing sensibility (sensibility capital such as forms of art and education, and the medical humanities) as in the hands of the few rather than the many. In other words, sensibility is still open to democratising. In the purely aesthetic realm, works of art do not simply appear as autonomous products received by a naïve public, but are produced within "modes of perception and regimes of emotion, categories that identify them, thought patterns that categorize and interpret them" (ibid.) as well as within material modes of production owned by large corporations such as pharmaceutical industries. Just as art/efacts and "taste" in art are shaped by a material infrastructure such as galleries and their sponsors, so industrially generated advertising, marketing, and packaging shape the fabric of modes of perception in a prescription culture.

The wealthiest living English artist Damien Hirst has famously turned pharmaceuticals and related apparatus (such as cabinets displaying pills) into art forms, reminding us that such pills as objects have aesthetic qualities within a Minimalist frame. The review below (artsy.net/artist-series/damien-hirst-pills-and-medicine) suggests that Hirst's pill installations "can be interpreted as a metaphor for the healing power of art". But this is a little corny. I don't think Hirst believes in art primarily as a healing force, but more as a disruptive presence, producing symptom (anxiety and confusion, uncertainty) and this, paradoxically, is precisely why people take recreational drugs – to disrupt their level lives:

> Famously obsessed with morbid subject matter, Damien Hirst first incorporated pharmaceuticals into his work in his 1980s "Medicine Cabinet" series, using old prescriptions found in the bathroom of his recently deceased grandmother. For this series, Hirst arranged the medicine according to their function on the human body—from migraine pills on the top shelf to foot cream on the bottom. In the years since, Hirst has made outsized sculptures of candy-colored pills …, as well as immersive installations that make the viewer feel like they've entered a working pharmacy. … Perhaps most admired is *The Void* (2000), a mammoth glass shelf containing single pills arranged in a perfect grid. "I think it's like the best piece I've ever made," Hirst said of the installation.
>
> *(Source: patreon.com)*

The topic of the regulation of mood through prescribed medications is of great interest to medical students. However, they tend to be introduced to this topic in a highly mechanical and literal way – through a reductive pharmacology, noting how drugs work instrumentally for generalised populations. The politics and aesthetics – the production and distribution of sensibility and insensibility and forms of resistance to this production – are rarely discussed but make for excellent content within a medical humanities curriculum. The students' text for the study of prescriptions is again the national formulary – pharmaceutical reference books produced nationally containing instrumental information and advice on prescribing, and on pharmacology related to populations, such as the BNF and the United States Pharmacopeia and the National Formulary (USP–NF).

Such formularies do not address individual responses, tastes, and tolerances; the contexts in which drugs are prescribed; whether they "work"; how they might be abused; the transformation of such drugs into guiding metaphors; and whether they become habitual and naturalised, or part of a cultural fabric. Such contextual insights are provided by artists, academics, journalists, and contemporary novelists. If medical students are lucky, they will discuss issues of prescription behaviour beyond technical knowledge of the drugs that are prescribed mainly by GPs and psychiatrists. But their education in this field normally revolves around a good deal of rote learning based on a drug formulary. Such a compendium of drugs and their effects is again written like a car manual. There are no patient case studies – indeed human presence appears to be excluded from the formulary that provides only technical or instrumental descriptions of the drugs, their main effects, and side effects. Also, the drugs themselves are described in terms of flat affect, although of course many of them produce strong affective responses in patients. The style of the formulary as a text is then an interesting study, returning us to the power of linguistics and semiotics as key facets of the medical humanities. "Flat affect" is no style at all and must not be confused with deadpan humour or minimalism, both of which have, rather, flat-packed a good deal of affect into their high-fidelity artefacts.

Where the formulary resists literary analysis, as it is more like a shopping list, contemporary literature is a powerful entry route into understanding prescription culture. Introducing medical students to the writers and literature discussed in this chapter, for example, and opening this up for critical discussion in intensive small group settings extends students' education, providing a counterpoint to the literal pharmacology that they learn. In conversation with GPs and psychiatrists on placements, students can further develop an understanding of, and insights into, prescribing behaviour or doctors' performances under stress. But it is in conversation with patients that students may best develop insight into prescription culture, and the creative writing associated with this culture detailed below fleshes out this understanding and insight. Again, *You Tube* has a raft of examples of patients talking about their relationships with prescription drugs that includes discussion of lifestyle, habits, identity, withdrawal, disorder, and differing drug "personalities" or identities. This is a rich source of educational material for the medical humanities.

Drugs as characters: American pharma-literature

During the early noughties, a small number of high-profile novels, particularly from North American authors, constituted a sub-genre of "prescription culture" books, where references to anti-anxiety and anti-depressant drugs were common. Such prescription drugs were part of the everyday fabric of people's lives, constituting animated objects, again ascribed personalities while their effects, paradoxically, appeared to erase distinctive personality traits from their users. For example, in his quasi-autobiographical novel *Lunar Park*, Bret Easton Ellis (2005: 10) goes shopping in his gentrified, suburban neighbourhood. It features "gourmet food stores, a first-class cheese shop, a row of patisseries, [and] a friendly pharmacist who filled my Klonopin and Xanax prescriptions". On Main Street anywhere, such drug transactions are happening in broad daylight. Some involve drugs for pre-school age children such as Ritalin, for control of attention deficit and hyperactivity. Most are for adults who do not need psychiatric intervention or hospitalisation, but are the "worried well", working long hours, possibly unhappy, certainly anxious. And many of these drugs, such as Xanax for control of free-floating anxiety, are designed to engineer wellbeing – mainly stabilising moods considered manic, or elevating moods considered depressive.

Later, Ellis (ibid.: 159) describes taking his six-year-old stepdaughter and 11-year-old son to a party. In the car, the girl "took a small canister and started popping Skittles into her mouth and throwing her head back as if they were prescription pills". "Why are you eating your candy that way, honey?" asks Ellis. "Because this is how Mommy does it when she's in the bathroom" replies the girl. Once they arrive at the party, Ellis "started noticing that all the kids were on meds (Zoloft, Luvox, Clexa, Paxil) that caused them to move lethargically and speak in affectless monotones" (ibid.: 161). One parent comments that his son is:

> "taking methylphenidate" – Adam pronounced it effortlessly – "even though it really hasn't been approved for kids under six," and then he went on about […] attention-deficit/hyperactivity disorder, which naturally led the conversation to the 7.5 milligrams of Ritalin administered three times a day.
>
> *(ibid.: 201)*

Note Ellis' use of "naturally". There is no moral tone in Ellis' report; indeed, his exact observation suggests if anything, coming to terms with the apparently inevitable. Prescription culture has become naturalised and normalised. Woven into the fabric of everyday living, prescription culture is apparently freed from the shackles of Big Pharma-led medicine, and largely from the illegal "street" drug trade. Prescription culture is part of sophisticated middle-class living promising better living through chemistry.

In a review of *Lunar Park*, Thomas (2005) notes that pharmaceuticals pervade the book. But the pharmaceutical work goes beyond content to pervade style. Conversation specifies "7.5 milligrams of Ritalin administered three times a day", speaking in the instrumental tones of the various drug formularies that inform the prescribing behaviour of doctors, such as the BNF, introduced earlier. But now the instrumental tone is partly parodied and used ironically, becoming a stylistic tool. The instrumentalism of the medical world is kidnapped by an educated lay public and aestheticised, made cool. Flat tone and flat personality signify a kind of effortlessness in life that is the new cool. It is, in part, a reborn aesthetic of minimalism, where surfaces signify depth. It is the 1950s "cool jazz" ethic of the West Coast: California cool.

While trade names for drugs may differ, the text styles of these formal "drug bibles" or formularies are identical. Where the formulary becomes the style of conversation adopted by Ellis' characters, it acts as a simulacrum preceding and forming reality. Further, while the text ostensibly describes symptoms to be cured, it comes to model such symptoms, inscribing rather than describing through the same "affectless monotones" and laconic styles as the medically doped children at the party. The conventional formulary is absorbed into a hip culture without real knowledge of its content or meaning, that, as noted, remains as capital of the medical world and pharmaceutical industry. In this way, both cognitive (informational) and emotional (wisdom and meaning) capital is captured from the medical world and re-distributed amongst a knowledgeable lay population as it is simultaneously captured and re-distributed by a criminal, fringe, and street culture. The point of this hip-ness is to remain aloof and uncritical, to dis-engage with an all-knowing smile, or smirk.

As this middle-class, educated appropriation of aspects of the medico-pharmaceutical culture took root in the early noughties, so *The Guardian* newspaper (Boseley 2006) carried a front-page headline: "Ritalin heart attacks warning urged after 51 deaths in US". The article warned of a statistically small chance that drugs prescribed for ADHD may increase risk of death from a heart attack. Ritalin and similar drugs are amphetamine-based and raise blood pressure. A handful of children have died this way in the UK since methylphenidate hydrochloride has been used to treat ADHD. The article goes on to say that two million prescriptions for drugs treating ADHD are written every month in the US. Over 30,000 prescriptions a month were written in the UK in 2005. By 2014, ADHD had grown to become the most common behavioural disorder in the UK, affecting 2–5% of school-aged children and young people (nhs.uk/conditions/attention-deficit-hyper-activity-disorder/Pages/Introduction.aspx). ADHD is now often referred to as "hyperkinetic disorder". Between 2016 and 2019, six million children in the USA were diagnosed with ADHD. Global prevalence is currently 5% for children and adolescents age less than 18. This surely constitutes a drug epidemic.

The Guardian article goes on to say that, however, "In the UK, nobody knows how many people are on the drugs, which are licensed for children as young as six – although there are reports of them being given to children as young as three". By 2014, as data were collected, 1.5% or just over 132,000 children and young people, 1.6% or about 70,000 children, and 1.4% or about 62,000 young people were diagnosed as having "severe ADHD" in the UK (http://www.youngminds.org.uk/train-ing_services/policy/mental_health_statistics). The National Institute for Health and Clinical Excellence (NICE) guidelines on ADHD (2009) (nice.org.uk/niceme-dia/pdf/adhdfullguideline.pdf) notes that a 1986 estimate of incidence of ADHD in the UK of 0.5 children per 1,000 rose to more than 3 per 1,000 of children actually receiving medication for ADHD by the late 1990s – a six-fold increase. In the USA during the same period, incidence rose from 12 per 1,000 to 35 per 1,000 – a threefold increase, but from a much higher base. Current UK figures suggest that 5% of adolescents and children suffer from ADHD (adhduk.co.uk).

This suggests opposite readings: either ADHD is a biological condition whose epidemiology was not fully understood but is now unfolding, or ADHD is a socially constructed condition and then cultural differences in diagnoses would be expected. As a socially constructed condition, we can venture that ADHD is wholly or partly shaped by the drug companies who provide Ritalin, Focalin, and so forth, amphetamines that "treat" the condition, or contain it. Whatever the case, mental health epidemics such as the rise in incidence of ADHD must be understood more widely than the somatic to include cultural factors, and then may also be understood through medical humanities interventions. The status of ADHD as socially constructed is echoed in a Big Pharma spoof by the Australian artist Justine Cooper in her parody advertising campaign for a fictional medication, first shown in New York City in 2007 (https://en.wikipedia.org/wiki/Havidol). Cooper's "Havidol" – a play on "have it all" – was a fictional drug for a spoof psychological condition: Dysphoric Social Attention Consumption Deficit Anxiety Disorder (DSACDAD). Havidol was further given a technical name: "avafynetyme", or "have a fine time". The American author Jonathan Franzen's (2001) novel *The Corrections* – discussed below – echoes this parody in inventing a range of fictional "optimisers", as tailored lifestyle-enhancing drugs.

The respectable use of prescription medicine is no secret, then. Accounts such as the *Guardian*'s are matched by regular scandals as the side effects of drugs emerge, and nobody is surprised to learn that drug companies are making huge profits. Yet any doctor can testify to the public's demand for this grown up "candy", in a world where so many are stressed, depressed and vulnerable. Again, a scan through the host of *You Tube* video confessions, primarily by young people, will attest to how complex this issue is (e.g. youtube.com/watch?v=ji0hg1LduU8). Many of these confessional videos concern withdrawal symptoms that outweigh the severity of the symptoms that were supposedly treated by the drug prescriptions in the first place.

But the writer Brett Easton Ellis unfolds a subtler diagnosis of prescription culture in *Lunar Park*. As much quasi-anthropological as literary, his deadpan life story shows medicine to be a privileged currency of family life. It binds relationships together, defining obligation, duty, guilt, and love. This can be summarised in the moment when Ellis unexpectedly restores a relationship with a girlfriend of 12 years previous, along with their son and her daughter by another relationship. "The summer", he says, was spent "getting acquainted with the wide array of meds the kids were on (stimulants, mood stabilizers, the antidepressant Lexapro, the Adderall for attention-deficit/hyperactivity disorder and various other anticonvulsants and antipsychotics that had been prescribed)" (Ellis 2005: 42). Even the household dog is on "meds" after a spell in canine behavioural therapy. The dog therapist had "prescribed Clomicalm, which was basically puppy Prozac". But a side effect of this drug, "compulsive licking", had kicked in, and the dog was now taking "a kind of canine Paxil [...] the same medication Sarah [his 6 year old stepdaughter] was on, which we all thought was extremely distressful" (ibid.: 47)!

Grotesque though the sight of their dog's compulsion may be, the family is principally worried by the fact that dog and child share the same prescription. Roles must be preserved in this carefully assembled family unit and getting to know each other's "meds" is part of their commitment to each other's happiness. Indeed, identities are now intimately linked with those "meds" and the (private and expensive) family physician is enrolled as part of the extended family, a kind of benevolent aunt or uncle promising sweets for all.

Prescriptions, particularly for children, emerge in this literature to offer contemporary rites of passage as normalised, where the illegal drug taking of adolescents and the complicit "convenience store" pharmaceutical industry facilitate this convenience. McGough and colleagues (2004) describe "extended-release capsules" for ADHD favoured by physicians because of "increased convenience". The extended-release form of dexmethylphenidate has the trade name of Focalin, promising increased focus. In the USA, the most prescribed of this group of drugs is Adderall, which is not licensed in the UK, but the three brands which are licensed conjure images of their promised effects: Ritalin = right/align, Concerta = in concert, and Equasym = equal/symmetrical. What is out of kilter must be adjusted. But adjusted to what? "Normalcy" seems like a mild form of depression, a dullness – or blankness – in itself. Anomie or alienation.

Doctors and healthcare professionals are widely consulted to suggest such snappy trade names. They thus contribute to powerful metaphors of what parents wish from their children, what partners expect from each other, perhaps precisely because they are semiotically so facile. "Focalin" echoes the "alignment" suggestions of Ritalin. A popular drug for male erectile dysfunction is called "Muse" (she can make you rise to the occasion), an appetite suppressant treating obesity is Reductil (she shrinks your needs), an anti-depressant aimed specifically at women is Lustral (implying that you regain far more than your shine), and so forth. This is the new theophany – the parade of gods and goddesses in pill form. Our forms of learning are indeed "socio-material".

We can find a precise analogy to the Lustral plot in Jonathan Franzen's (2001) saga of nuclear family implosion, *The Corrections*. Here a parallel between recreational drugs and the medication of the elderly is the joke. A hopeless literature lecturer loses it all for a weekend of sex with one of his students, who brings along a supply of what she calls "Mexican A". Later, we find out his elderly mother Enid is prescribed the same thing by a doctor on her retiree cruise ship, when she finds herself insomniac with worry over her Parkinson's disease-afflicted husband – only here it goes by the name of Aslan, after C.S. Lewis' redemptive lion in Narnia. When Edith asks what "ASLAN® CruiserTM" does, the doctor replies "Absolutely nothing, if you are in perfect mental health. However, let's face it, who is"? He explains that "Aslan provides a state-of-the-art factor regulation. The best medications now approved for American use are like two Marlboros and a rum-and-Coke, by comparison". Enid asks if it is an antidepressant, to which he replies: "Crude term. 'Personality optimizer' is the phrase preferred" (ibid.: 369–70). Manufactured by a company named *Farmacopea*, Aslan's plentiful varieties are each optimised for a particular activity or mental state. Besides Aslan Basic there is Aslan Ski, Aslan Hacker, Aslan Performance Ultra, Aslan Teen, Aslan Club Med, Aslan Golden Years, and Aslan California. The company also plans to bring several other blends to market, namely Aslan Exam Buster, Aslan Courtship, Aslan White Nights, Aslan Reader's Challenge, Aslan Connoisseur Class, and several others. The drug is "not available" in America. When Enid asks if she can get in her home-town of St. Jude he advises her to get her Aslan from Mexico.

More chilling than Franzen's spoof, prescription culture is most thoroughly charted in the late David Foster Wallace's 1996 sprawling novel *Infinite Jest*. This darkly comic work centres on the narrative of a videotape said to be so entertaining that it guarantees compulsive viewing leading to loss of desire for any other activity. Viewers die happily watching the tape in endless repetition. The parallels with prescription drugs discussed here are obvious. Part of the novel is set in a halfway house for recovering addicts. Wallace uses this setting to explore some of the contradictions inherent in the culture of prescribing, including the recreational use of such drugs – in Wallace's phrase, "abusing prescribed meds". But where Wallace talks of "abuse" he is being descriptive not prescriptive. In one scene, a woman has been admitted to the "psych ward" of a hospital after an overdose and is being interviewed by the psychiatrist. She starts in a matter-of-fact way: "I took a hundred-ten Parnate, about thirty Lithonate capsules, some old Zoloft" and then, "I took everything I had in the world"; or, the drugs took everything, consumed her whole being. The doctor's reply is flat, technical, missing the point of her admission to total annihilation: "You really must have wanted to hurt yourself, then, it seems" (ibid.: 70).

She continues with a vivid description of the overdose in which we sense that she has sought rebirth within the suicide attempt:

> They said downstairs the Parnate made me black out. It did a blood pressure thing. My mother heard the noises upstairs and found me she said down on my side chewing the rug in my room. My room's shag-carpeted. She said I was on the floor flushed red and all wet like when I was a new-born; she said she thought at first she hallucinated me as a newborn again. On my side all red and wet.
>
> *(Ibid.: 70)*

The doctor's response to this vivid memory is merely informative (also giving Wallace an opportunity to show off his technical interests):

> A hypertensive crisis will do that. It means your blood pressure was high enough to have killed you. Sertraline in combination with an MAOI will kill you, in

enough quantities. And with the toxicity of that much lithium besides, I'd say you were pretty lucky to be here right now.

She tries to re-engage the memory of the near-death: "My mother sometimes thinks she's hallucinating", but Wallace has the doctor bundling on through with weakly disguised prescription: "Sertraline, by the way, is the Zoloft you kept instead of discarding as instructed when changing medications". She has one more attempt to engage him affectively even adding a rhetorical question: "She says I chewed a big hole out of the carpet. But who can say"? But the psychiatrist's attention is already elsewhere – focused on his freebie drug company pens in fact: "The doctor chose his second-finest pen from the array in his white coat's breast pocket and made some sort of note on Kate Gompert's new chart" (ibid.: 70, 71). These descriptive and then weak prescriptive gestures finally become inscriptions: writing out and re-inscribing the patient's identity. Wallace himself became intimate with mental health pharmaceuticals as he struggled with depression throughout his adult life and moved back and forth between drug treatment regimes. He tragically committed suicide in 2008 at the age of 46 at the peak of his writing powers. For Wallace, prescription drugs seemed to help to keep his depression at bay, but eventually the "black dog" overwhelmed him. We suspect that writing – and Wallace was amongst the most talented fiction and non-fiction writers of his generation – offered the main therapy in Wallace's life. Metaphor kept him alive.

Doctors in general write in linear, instrumental, and non-literary ways through prescribing, where the act of writing a drug prescription is also the inscription of identity through a "habitus" (Bourdieu 1977) or typical pattern of practice. Such prescribing then carries over the complications and contradictions inherent to the drug – particularly side effects – to the identity of the patient. Ironically, significant numbers of young women are found to self-harm when taking Seroxat, a drug that promised to reduce psychological harm, thus transforming the cure into symptom. This has been read as an instrumental side effect of the drug. Similarly, drug companies admit the possible occurrence of what they term "paradoxical effects", in the control of "hyperactivity". In the BNF, a listed side effect (albeit "rarely occurring") for Ritalin is "hyperactivity"! The most reported side effect of extended-release Focalin is its inverse, insomnia. Kids then need another drug to help them sleep: Ellis is informed blankly by his son that his friend "Ashton took a Zyprexa and then fell asleep. … Well, I suggest you take one too, buddy, because tomorrow's a school day" (Ellis 2005: 69). Zyprexa is an antipsychotic, causing drowsiness.

In prescription culture, the relationship between natural life and prescribed chemical life becomes increasingly blurred. But these writers do not protest. Much like the chemical hall of mirrors with which they jest, they mimic the bad faith of their self-harming characters. Their drawling satires refuse to confess their addictions, rather, laconically describing their own pleasure-pain complicity in the synthetic reality of prescription culture.

Deconstructing drugs

Brett Easton Ellis, David Foster Wallace and Jonathan Franzen are often seen as second-generation postmodernists. Along with others such as Jay McInerney, Rick Moody, Tama Janowitz, and J. Robert Lennon, they perpetuate an urban knowing and savvy reflexivity that sees through (in both senses) the institutionalised games of insight that have come to characterise contemporary life. Unlike earlier writers who have explored the social construction of drug culture, they undermine the markers for even an ironic morality on drugs.

Pointing out the continuities between illegal and legal drug taking is not new, any more than accounting for the ordinariness of "madness". But these writers do not romanticise mental instability as an alternative to prescribed drugs, as Ronald Laing, David Cooper and the anti-psychiatry movement did in the 1960s. Nor do they romanticise pharmaceuticals, or explicitly condone the abuse of prescribed drugs, as did the Beat Generation of the 1950s and early 1960s (Alex Trocchi, Allen Ginsberg, William Burroughs), and the Acid Generation of the mid-1960s onwards ("Gonzo" writers inspired by Hunter S. Thompson), who tend to write hysterically. Even compared to the satirical surrealism of the first generation of postmodernists, J.G. Ballard, Thomas Pynchon and Don DeLillo, these information age writers are more detached, mirroring the plain descriptions of the pharmaceutical world itself.

It is the medical formulary's sober semiotics, instrumental listing, and clipped voice with which the chroniclers of prescription culture play. Coolly witnessing the world, yet simultaneously exaggerating its detail, they implode the moral bounds of earlier postmodern drug reverie. "N.B. narr tone here mxmly flat/ affectless/ distant/dry", where there is "no discernable endorsement of cliché", remarks David Foster Wallace (1996: 33, 34) in a short story titled "Adult World", echoing the style markers of Samuel Beckett. But here is a discernable cliché: that of clinical formulae. The central character in Wallace's short story "The Depressed Person" is introduced simply through her anti-depressant drugs' history, as a flat list: "Paxil, Zoloft, Prozac, Tofranil, Welbutrin, Elavil, Metrazol ... Parnate both with and without lithium salts, Nardil both with and without Xanax". This can be read as a satire on the reductionist style of the case history taught to medical students in every medical school where the patient is boiled down to hard tack symptoms, transmitted with flat affect to produce further objectification. Here is the advice from Weill Cornell Medical College (weill.cornell.edu/education/curriculum/third/med_gui_cas.html):

> Summarize the case: this is important! The summary should include a few well-crafted sentences, perhaps 3-5 in all. A concise, accurate summary shows that you have grasped the essentials of the case and can distill the clinical data into its essence.

The fiction writers we discuss here bolster this disembodied hyper-realism with pseudo-erudition and the (ab)use of academic trappings, such as Rick Moody's

(2002) quotations from historians of American Puritanism – italicised, suggesting sarcastic emphasis. David Foster Wallace (1996) literally attaches pages of footnotes on the drugs his characters navigate, and in the process personifies the drugs, thus emphasising their role in identity construction, such as "Oxycodone hydrochloride w/ acetaminophen, C-II Class, Du Pont Pharmaceuticals" (ibid.: 996); or the post-operative pain killer, "Ketorolac tromethamine, a non-narcotic analgesic" personified as "little more than Motrin with ambition" (ibid.: 1076). At least we have an innovative metaphor here. Substituting drug discourse for character, quotation for expression, they usually avoid depth of metaphor, preferring the metonymic technique of offering part for whole, or, we might say, symptom for aetiology. Moody muses that lists themselves are suggestive of an ethical paralysis, but one which he dryly witnesses without being able to stop – a sure sign of addiction: "The list itself, the catalog, as a journalistic gesture, generates further lists. In fact, the list itself becomes a frequent compositional trope of murderers …" (ibid.: 223).

Thus, it appears that these writers deconstruct prescription culture simply by citing it. But, of course, there is a familiar aesthetic at work here. The ouroboric worm eats itself from the tail and emerges re-born as a simulacrum of a style: that of the drug formulary. The aesthetic is also in the trimmings. Who but Wallace might conceive of the descriptor "little more than Motrin with ambition"? This is a postmodern aesthetic, and one drawn on by Damien Hirst's pill installations described earlier. The artefact (and of course Marcel Duchamp was the forerunner of this) is presented as it is, as an ironic gesture. But it is presented in cultural context: the latrine, bicycle wheel, or hatstand in a gallery setting, demanding that such objects be considered for their aesthetic and not functional worth. Who could improve on the aesthetic of the manufactured pill as aesthetically pleasing variations on the sphere? For the sphere is the origin of "pill", the Latin *pillula* used to describe a round ball in medieval times, akin to a bullet. Now we have pharmaceutical magic bullets. Brett Easton Ellis' little girl "pops" her Skittles imitating her mother popping pills as an aesthetic gesture (necessarily ethically and politically troubling).

Moody's moods

In Rick Moody's (2002) memoir, *The Black Veil*, Moody charts his youthful ambition to self-destruct through drug-taking and drinking, weaving this alongside the story of his forbear Joseph Moody, a 17th-century preacher who wore a black face veil through life in shame of having killed a friend as a child. Moody's dry conclusion that "concealment is necessary to identity" (ibid.: 298) thus checks his own confession of shame at addictions and breakdown. It also checks any acknowledgement of his therapists, who are glimpsed as either sharks or fools:

> Beyond stories, my principal interest in these expensive consultations with the mental health professional was not the back and forth of conversation, to which I offered as little as possible, but rather *the drugs*, because, by virtue of the

unexplained panic event, I had been given a certain prescription, and I carried the vial of it with me wherever I went.

(ibid.: 139)

Later, attending a rehabilitation programme as partner to his equally alcoholic girlfriend, he is pulled aside by a counsellor "in her late thirties, with a red bob", whose sweaters were "*excessively colourful*" (ibid.: 178):

It was naïve to have failed to see that I was going to look *appetizing* to the employees at the rehabilitation center, especially when my mental health professional back home, in a strangely paranoid outburst, had warned me to be on the alert for this very possibility. *These AA people will try to convert you.*

(ibid.: 179)

Even when he spontaneously checks himself into a psychiatric hospital and stops drinking, Moody maintains his arid performance. Rather, and in this way, he also marks out the deconstructive approach to drugs, he suggests that poststructuralist "Theory" had been his true turning point:

in junior year, I took a couple of film courses in the department known as *semiotics* … This brought me, at last, to 'Foundation of the Theory of Signs,' or Semiotics 12. *Where the school of deconstruction welcomed its fresh prospects.*

(ibid.: 95)

This period was near Moody's twentieth birthday "and a number of crises were in the midst of their germination". He had broken up with a long-term girlfriend and fell in with "not one but two mercurial, dark, undependable women". The first introduced him to cocaine. He also started taking large quantities of a "prescription medicine" that "a friend … referred to as *Australian quaaludes*. They were probably strong anti-histamines, not much more". However,

Taken in large enough doses […] or combined with beer, they made my friend's customers, myself among them, thoroughly confused. I experienced my first regular blackouts on these pills, and whole days were lost. Or I came to at some party having shredded articles of my clothing and talking like a reptile.

(ibid.: 96)

When his second "mercurial, dark, undependable" woman ditched him, Moody "decided to take *all* the quaaludes, with some Jack Daniel's", which he refers to as "my *unconvincing suicide attempt*" (ibid.: 96). He remembers taking maybe 15 pills and then falling asleep, waking 12 or 14 hours later to realise that he was "*missing my discussion section of semiotics*". The set reading is Michel Foucault's (1991) *Discipline and Punish*. Moody arrives at the class but

> I put my head down on my desk and went to sleep. I didn't wake again until the stirring of the rest of the class at lunchtime. You'd think a *conversion*, a battering of the heart, couldn't possibly have firm tread on such lassitude, but sometimes conversion is like pines that grow on glacial outcroppings.
>
> *(ibid.: 97)*

Moody goes on to describe the trajectory of this surprisingly rooted *conversion*: "when I had expelled the quaaludes in me, *Discipline and Punish* looked entirely new". He suddenly *saw* Foucault's "extremely artful and generous" theory about the displacement of sovereign power by capillary power, where "*The body is directly involved in a political field; power relations have an immediate hold upon it; they invest it, mark it, train it, torture it, force it to carry out tasks, to perform ceremonies, to emit signs*". The body is both disciplined and resists governance in new ways. Importantly,

> The theories of Foucault […] seemed to have […] more in common with novels than with the dry social theory that I had found in my philosophy classes. And it was this novelistic dimension that kindled in me the *zealotry of the newly converted.*
>
> *(ibid.: 97)*

Theory becomes a drug.

For Rick Moody, conversion to the new semiotics comes to displace his suicidal wishes. The deep semiotics of theory replaces the surface semiotics of mood design by chemistry. Moody's "conversion" centrally involves his insight into the power of Foucault's suggestion that the replacement of sovereign power by capillary power does not represent the progress ("freedom from") claimed by liberalism, but rather offers a pervading governmentality. This translates our prescription drugs into pharmaceutical prisons, ongoing forms of surveillance and control. Where, again, moral injunctions or imperatives may be disguised as invitations to freedoms ("Enjoy!", "Have a nice day"!), supposedly liberating prescription drugs may then become literally prescriptive, a cultural injunction. But this insight does not in fact stop his drug habit, which is merely deferred. Moody's post-ironic response is to live that injunction out, to explore its terrible shame, to refuse to confess to what he suggests, in the end, is American culture itself.

BNF-rictus

From this perspective, we might interpret these writers' refusal to moralise as a protest – against prescription culture's own hypocritical plot of conversion and cure.

Their apparent detachment offers commentary without prescribing, thus smuggling in critique at the level of style which they do not offer at the level of plot. Ironically, then, as they themselves "write out prescriptions", medical handbooks such as the BNF come into relief as exercises in the hyper-real of their own.

The BNF, designedly instrumental, is also a descriptive catalogue that strains to bracket out the contexts in which the various consumptions of its contents (or drugs as main characters) take place. From its terse notices of "contra-indications" and "side effects", in the people-ness landscape of its passive tense, and in appendices where its classifications blur, we sense repressed scenes of parents organising their kids' medications, or students' swapping of drug stories. The following, under the heading of "Borderline Substances", is appended to the entry on Zyprexa discussed above:

> In certain conditions some foods (and toilet preparations) have characteristics of drugs and the Advisory Committee on Borderline Substances advises as to the circumstances in which such substances may be regarded as drugs. Prescriptions issued in accordance with the Committee's advice and endorsed 'ACBS' will normally not be investigated.

The absence of a human(e) voice – a main feature of instrumentalism – in the text of the BNF reflects the search for perfection through new levels of biotechnological intervention, but in its marginal appendices and footnotes, we glimpse its own borderlines. The BNF acts as a rictus superego, a smiling know-all and moraliser, Freud's infamous "absent presence" that frames invitation as imperative (again, "Enjoy!", "Have a Nice Day!", leading us to face the world with a Klonopin rictus, a Duchenne smile, empty ecstasy). There is no reflexive voice – but simply, again, flat prescription. Its monologue describes a world in which the simulacrum has come to precede the real, or the map displaces the territory.

The deconstructive novelists considered above chart their responses to the creeping pharmaceutical culture in the backhanded manner of Jacques Derrida's philosophy, attempting not so much to judge as to both violently differentiate and tenderly defer. In this way, such deconstructive writing does not offer a "cure" for prescription culture at all, but an exaggeration of its symptoms, the diagnosis of a diagnosis, the double "writing out" of its paradoxical effects. However, we argue that this rather tortuous approach does have benefits.

The value of literary deconstruction in understanding health interventions

We have explored a literary rather than sociological response to the prescription of mood-altering drugs as a "health" intervention because we consider that literature plumbs the social unconscious in a different and powerful way. The novels we have discussed deconstruct the objectivity of medical texts and expose the contrary injunction to "be happy!" that sustains prescription culture, but they do this in the form of imaginative symptoms, rather than explications, of a condition that they themselves share.

No doubt many readers will find that these writers overemphasise the determining aspects of "prescription" as habitus. The synthesising research by Pound and colleagues (2005: 1) on patients' actual behaviour in relation to prescriptions reveals there is "widespread caution about taking medicines", that they do not just "accept their medicines [...] passively", but "actively, or ... (choose to) ... reject them". This is as true in relation to mood-altering drugs as it is with others, and, moreover, is also the case in the United States as well as in Britain, which not only has an exceptionally high consumption rate but the highest drug prices in the world, towards which most patients are making co-payments. "The main reason why people do not take their medicines as prescribed is not because of failings in patients, doctors or systems, but because of concerns about the medicines themselves" (ibid.: 1).

The style of the deconstructive writers discussed above models the paradox (and double bind) of the *pharmakon* – the drug as both "poison" and "cure". Jacques Derrida (1993), deconstruction's inventor, if it can be said to have one, argued in "The Rhetoric of Drugs" that we should stop scapegoating drug-taking, noting the artificial line drawn between the *pharmakon* as remedy (*prescription pharmaceuticals* are social, authentic, natural, demanding, and productive), and poison (*illicit drugs* are solitary, fantastical, unnatural, effortless, and unproductive). Boothroyd (2000) argues that deconstruction presents the possibility of an alternative thinking of the relation to "drugs". If we take Boothroyd's case to refer to prescription culture as well as recreational drug culture, and then to include anti-depressant, anti-anxiety, and ADHD medications, it raises very important questions about prescribing as a "health" intervention:

> [D]rugs may be taken *otherwise* – in a sense for which there is as yet no concept, on the basis of a non-authoritarian, deregulated understanding of their *multiple* effects, in *several* senses. In other words, the force of the dominant drug rhetorics may be countered by the deratiocinatory force of a reinscribed notion of drugs. Could there be a *measure* for drugs, unfettered, for example, by such rhetorics as those of authenticity and inauthenticity, of health and illness, of use and abuse, etc.?
>
> *(ibid.: 58)*

This characteristically displacing quote suggests in fact that deconstruction can be *equated* with drug taking, for both undo notions of truth and order which are naturalised in prescription culture.

Deconstructing arbitrary distinctions between medicine and drugs, then, has little to say about the free will lost in addiction, and nothing about the evidence of patients' control over, or even rejection of, prescription drugs. But this is not its point, nor its usefulness to those working in the everyday of healthcare. Rather, it is precisely its doubt about individual agency that so powerfully dramatises prescription culture's micro-disciplining effects and the wider dissolution of a belief in free will that permits it. A warning and a seduction in one, it exemplifies the same psychology that, without self-consciousness, offers doctors (who offer patients) the National Formulary.

Coda: development of a humanities-based formulary

It is not enough to simply point out that there are striking similarities between the flat affect of the BNF (or any other, similar pharmaceutical formulary) and the stylised hyperrealism of the postmodern novelists whose work we discuss above. What should be done about this that may improve medical education with a view to a knock-on effect on patient care and safety? The argument above is that such postmodern writers, who have a cultivated and developed technique of presenting the world as marketplace shaped partly by Big Pharma interests (Law 2006), do so in a highly detached and very articulate, wry manner that is gendered male. In striking contrast, many of the confessional *You Tube* videos show young women who are struggling to articulate their symptoms and the side effects of drugs often in claustrophobic confessions.

The smart postmodern writers catalogued in this chapter model an ironic style that is in part a deliberate attempt to recreate through literature a consciousness that in turn is shaped by regular use of antidepressants, anti-anxiety, and mood controlling drugs such as the amphetamine-based medications for ADHD. However, we also point out that such literature appears to have misplaced its heart, interested more in the cold mechanics of deconstructing society than in the warm art of constructing humane relations and activities. Feelings are not missing from such literature; it is just that these feelings tend to be ones of colder detachment and observation rather than warm attachment, empathy, and concern.

How might we respond in medical education, through the medical humanities, to the issues raised by this chapter? The introductory paragraphs in this book suggest that medical students appreciate the opportunity to discuss "prescription culture" beyond their technical knowledge of pharmacology and prescribing behaviour. The postmodern novels discussed above offer a unique way into prescription culture and an aspect of population medicine that invites students to read beyond the BNF, but, paradoxically, to draw textual parallels between the BNF and postmodern, deconstructive novels. But there is another step – to invite students to begin to construct an "alternative" or "critical" BNF.

Here is a challenge for medical educators interested in the humanities – how might we develop a limited electronic BNF (based, say on a few mood-altering drugs used regularly by GPs and psychiatrists) in which we do two things. First, we develop profiles of patients (case studies) that accompany the technical descriptions of drugs, their effects and side effects. At the heart of this part of the alternative formulary are patients' stories concerning their relationship to prescribed drugs. Indeed, as already noted, a bank of such visually enhanced stories is already available on *You Tube*. Here, mainly young people talk about their individual experiences with anti-depressants, anti-anxiety and other mood regulating and mood enhancing drugs. Many of these stories stress "regulation" over "enhancement".

Second, we can develop "character profiles" of the drugs themselves, treating them as active agents. The socio-material Actor-Network-Theory (ANT) (Bleakley 2014) is slowly becoming an influential model in medical education research and pedagogy, both as a conceptual framework and a research approach using ethnography. ANT proposes a radical symmetry between persons, ideas, and material artefacts where the latter are given agency. As noted earlier, Object-Oriented Ontology (Harman 2018) suggests a similar "flat ontology" model – a democracy of persons, living things, and artefacts. This is not hard to comprehend if we think of computers as extending our cognition and a variety of pharmaceuticals as extending our senses, affects, and cognitions or regulating potential disruptions. Developing a character profile of a drug in concert with a character profile of a patient gives a way for medical students to better imagine the potential interactions between persons and drugs, where the latter can act as allies or foes. The alternative formulary can then be developed as a mobile device application. The elements in the learning network for understanding more about prescription culture are then: novels such as those described in this chapter, patients with mental health issues related to prescribed anti-anxiety and anti-depressant drugs and/or *You Tube* confessional videos, a "living" mini *Critical Formulary* in which the drugs are not only described in functional terms, but case studies are provided to give a human face to the mechanics of the pharmacopoeia. This would be the medical humanities in action in medical education, serving to raise the productive metaphor count.

Acknowledgement

Parts of this chapter owe much to a previous collaboration with Professor Margaretta Jolly.

9

THE NARRATIVE TURN

Peary's shifting sea

In his novel *Ragtime*, E.L. Doctorow (1976: 67, 68) recounts the first expedition to the North Pole in 1909, led by Robert Peary and the African American sailor and explorer Matthew Henson. Peary, exhausted, suffering from frostbite, and destined to be the first to plant the American flag at the exact geographical spot,

> Lay on his stomach and with a pan of mercury and a sextant, some paper and a pencil, he calculated his position. It did not satisfy him. He walked further along the floe and took another sighting. This did not satisfy him. All day long Peary shuffled back and forth over the ice, a mile one way, two miles another, and made his observations. No one observation satisfied him. He would walk a few steps due north and find himself going due south. On this watery planet the sliding sea refused to be fixed.

Peary eventually planted the flag and took the obligatory photograph of his team. Peary's prize was challenged by Frederick Cook who claimed to have reached the North Pole a year earlier. After a good deal of wrangling, in 1911 the US Congress recognised Peary's claim, suspecting some fraud in Cook's account, whose moral compass was awry. Peary's shifting compass was of a different order, perhaps based on self-doubt. The fluid North Pole that Peary experienced may have been in his own hesitant mind, or it may have been a product of the way that the environment played with his senses.

Peary's perceived shifting North Pole on Doctorow's "sliding sea" will act here as a twin-barrelled metaphor for the uncertainty in medicine and medical education that the medical humanities face head on (here in the form of fiction rather

DOI: 10.4324/9781003383260-10

than fact), and from which they profit. This, rather than the bottom-line certainty demanded by biomedical discourse. And within the medical humanities, narrative-based medicine has claimed the ever-shifting ground of accounting for illness. For a story – it is claimed – is what an illness traces, where the account provided by the patient is surely central to the process of doctors re-telling those stories in technical terms as diagnoses. So far, so narrative medicine. Narrative approaches to medicine are now more or less synonymous with the medical humanities.

Simultaneously, as multiple narrativist approaches have gained a foothold and acquired hegemony within medical and health humanities, they have also energetically resisted, deflected, or subdued critique from within their own camps. More, as we expand on later, where narrative approaches are, by definition, time-based accounts, these have occluded space-based accounts typical of non-narrative lyrical poetry. Indeed, poetry has been suffocated by contemporary narrative medicine; or, narrative has wrested the territory from its erstwhile companion, poetry. In our view, the flag of narrative is often mis-planted in the field that is rightly lyric poetry's turf (Bleakley and Neilson 2021). An ideal situation is where narrative and poetry co-exist, neither bent on imperialism.

Time-based narrative medicine's occupation of the labile territory of the medical humanities is troublesome because there are other rich and longstanding approaches within the medical humanities (drawn from the visual arts, music, the performing arts, history, philosophy, anthropology, and so forth), many of which are space- and place-based. Setting out as a necessary foil to reductive biomedicine and instrumental ethics, narrative medicine has now outgrown its boots to the extent that the movement has lost sight of the limits to its powers. Proponents will claim that narrative medicine, above all, *works* as an essential part of patient care, a qualitative "parallel chart" to the patient's quantitative medical chart. But then, what "works" most obviously in the medical humanities is the pre-verbal or primal, the pre-narrative, as touch and comfort; alas, these all-too-human strategies do not create credentialling mills.

The use of narrative in medical education is not intrinsically problematic. One cannot ignore its potential value. After all, we needed story's leverage (in this case Doctorow's) and the power of metaphor to carry us to this point. Despite our gratitude to the power of story to create greater understanding and insight, we again point out that there is much reflexive critical work to be done within narrative-based medicine. Where, we ask, are the proponents of narrative medicine who pause in their tracks and closely scrutinise their claims? We have recently pursued extensive critical work in this respect (Bleakley and Neilson 2021, 2023).

E.L. Doctorow, above, illustrates in less than one paragraph the key elements of narrative or story: (1) there is a series of events unfolding over time that illustrates a developing plot leading to a climax; (2) there are characters who move that plot forwards; and (3) there is some form of denouement (from the French: "unplotting"), meaning a conclusion after the climax in the story where the complexities and entanglements of the plot are picked apart such that conflict is resolved.

Of course, there are endless deviations from this master plan that still leave the writing and the telling in the realm of "story", but with creative enhancements or deconstructions of the ideal framework. Vladimir Propp's (1968) classic analysis of folk tales describes 31 possible dimensions to a story's structure. Yet the dominant strains of narrative medicine tend to have little to say about these deviations, preferring as they do the tidiness of their model as it relates to manageable and digestible clinical encounters. We will touch on this later as this can illuminate medical concerns, drawing for example on Samuel Beckett's debriding of "story".

It is extraordinary how narrative medicine has gained a kind of Teflon exterior, batting off critics, while also short-circuiting the very critical faculties that it encourages through techniques such as "close reading", considered later. In this and the following chapter we engage in an act of "sly civility" as formulated by Homi Bhabha (2004). We adopt the signature technique of narrative studies to "close read" a quarter of a century of narrative medicine, thereby offering a critical review.

The narrative turn of the screw: narrative's seductive side

In a review of Peter Brooks' (2022) *Seduced by Story: The Use and Abuse of Narrative*, Jennifer Szalai (2022) says "Imagine taking in an orphaned baby bird, giving it food and shelter so that it could grow, and then one day it swoops down and attacks the family hamster". The devouring monster that "narrative" has become was first noticed by Brooks in 2000 when George Bush, then president-elect, was presenting members of his cabinet to the public, whence Bush referred to each of his appointees as having their own "story", such "stories" collectively explaining "what America is about". At that point, Brooks, says Szalai, lost the plot. A celebrated narratologist, Brooks saw that the focus of his academic work, the nourishment of a narrative sensibility, had become a hegemonic monster. His academic pursuit had become trivialised. Now, we have "mindless valorization of storytelling … inertly accepting the notion that all is story, and that the best story wins" (ibid.). Brooks does not throw the baby out with the bathwater however, where good narrative avoids "shoddy contrivance with heavy-handed manipulation" – the hallmark of political rhetoric.

Brooks' moment of realisation was a long time coming. "The narrative turn" was a phrase coined in the late 1970s to describe a new wave of critical thinking based on exploring and explaining phenomena as, and through, story. It was applied particularly to social sciences research, where dissatisfaction with the limitations of quantitative methods of research following experimental science models gave rise to qualitative methods of inquiry. Though stories remained harvested as data as per tradition, data were also reported in the literature through story devices (thereby increasing the standing or credibility of "narrative inquiry" as a quasi-science) (Bleakley 2005). The so-called "narrative turn" intensified in the late 1980s, in part due to the work of psychologist Jerome Bruner (1986) who popularised story as a means of forming and deepening identity, maintaining that we, as it were, "story" ourselves into being. In turn, narrative perspectives came to transform medical ethics. Whereas previous approaches were based on rules or principles (for example beneficence or doing good, non-maleficence or doing no harm, autonomy or giving freedom to an individual's voice, and justice or ensuring fairness) illustrated through case studies, narrative-based ethics focused on the case studies themselves as literary forms open to close reading. Cases were read as rhetorical "fictions" or "stories" constructed such that they illustrated specific arguments or perspectives made by narrativists (Chambers 1999).

Story implies fiction, or, in what we offer as a concentrated definition, invented events viewed from a particular perspective. The narrative turn in the discipline of history offers an instructive case. A major paradigm shift occurred where, previously, history had claimed factual, unbiased account from archival or artefactual evidence. Michel Foucault amongst others showed that history was neither linear nor "true", but perspectival. Archival evidence could be employed selectively to piece together a story representing the conditions of possibility for the emergence of a phenomenon such as "madness" or the birth of the medical "clinic".

The narrative turn in time became a question of what was wagging – tail, or dog? Bleakley (2005), as noted above, makes a distinction between stories as data (narrative-based research) and data as stories (scientific research claiming "truth" status, where in fact a narrative is spun, making the data relative). Where Barusch (2012) asks "when does story-telling become research?", Bleakley asks: "when does research become story-telling?" To look at a more popular case: the narrative turn in natural history is evident from the spate of television programmes spearheaded by the work of Sir David Attenborough. Here, animals and plants become characters in stories, usually grounded in the conflict metaphor, that nature is "red in tooth and claw". Functional, bottom-line Darwinian values dominate such programmes that are all about survival of the fittest in a world of scarce resources. Function trumps form, where an array of spectacular animals and plants are not viewed primarily for their self-display, their beauty, but for their predatory, territorial, or mating behaviour. The aesthetic spectacle is reduced through an optics of "survival of the fittest" to instrumental competition. Thus, the story told is not biological fact, but a human projection of conflict narrative (ultimately grounded in Homer's epic *The Iliad*). Yet how can animal or plant life consciously inhabit a temporally experienced universe with plot, characters, and genres? The effect of the narrative turn in this field has been to flatten the world into a human-centred site, a move with many negative consequences for humans, but more importantly for the planet.

The narrative turn discussed above came to medicine late in the game as a challenge to the dominance of biomedical science as the main frame for patient care. From the early 1990s onward, medicine's version of "fact" was ring-fenced as "evidence-based practice", a term coined by Gordon Guyatt in 1990 (Guyatt et al. 1992). In this tradition, recommended treatments are based on interpretations of what are perceived as the most powerful and valid research tools: double-blind, placebo-controlled clinical trials. Yet the applicability of such crowd-derived "facts" to individuals remained an open question, problematising the practice of medicine as an exclusive application of bioscience. As this book has stressed repeatedly, medicine is about marrying biomedical expertise with judgement about qualities.

Other disciplinary approaches are needed for the rigours of medical practice besides translation of bioscience as medicine draws on a range of value perspectives. Clearly, doctors attend not just to symptom complexes in a quasi-algorithmic fashion based in probabilities, but also to the patient's "story" as a qualitative event. Because taking (or better, receiving) a history is, conventionally speaking, the first step in the diagnostic process, there is a natural progression to expanding traditional medical practice to appreciate story. Perhaps because the applicability of narrative approaches was intuitive, and because of a general dissatisfaction on the part of patients and doctors both with the prevailing bioscientific mode of clinical practice, it was inevitable that narrative-based methods would be developed to enhance clinical practice (Neilson 2022). Medicine being such a strongly credentialed discipline, doctors were soon told that they could not rely on an intuitive grasp of listening to a patient's story, that they needed "narrative competence" to seriously address how stories could be part of medical reasoning (Charon 2006; Charon et al. 2016). This involved an appreciation of a quite limited form of narratology to understand issues such as the nature of discourse, structures of story, and the use of linguistic tropes such as metaphor.

Whence narrative in medicine?

It is worth looking at the history of the genesis of various kinds of narrative medicine, and at the conditions inspiring their development. The resistance movement to perceived biomedical reductionism had started slowly in the 1970s, gaining considerable traction two decades later. By 1994, faculty with expertise in literature were employed in one-third of medical schools in North America. Kathryn Montgomery Hunter (1991) – possessing an academic background in literature, but no clinical experience – and others, including Anne Hudson Jones, introduced literary perspectives to better understand the human face of medicine. Jones was the longstanding editor of the journal *Literature and Medicine* (itself established because of the resistance movement to the dominance of functional biomedicine). Such literary perspectives could be essentialised as focusing on qualities of language in clinical encounters. Montgomery Hunter's (ibid.: 193) premise was that doctors are not pure scientists, but "rational science-using" practitioners whose clinical reasoning is already grounded in a hermeneutic method involving close attention to cues and clues as a kind of interpretive "sleuthing". A literary demonstration of this idea comes in the way that Conan Doyle (a doctor himself) inscribed the investigative method of the fictional Sherlock Holmes.

Montgomery Hunter (ibid.; 2005) called her field of inquiry "Doctor's Stories", the title of her influential first book; while she termed the main practice in this field "The Narrative Structure of Medical Knowledge", her subtitle. Her focus was less on the doctor-patient interaction in terms of co-construction of stories (a framework later adopted by Rita Charon), but more on the clinical reasoning process as a meaning-making exercise grounded in narrative expertise. She launched a movement in North America that we now generally recognise as generic "narrative-based medicine". Kathryn Montgomery (2006) described this structure of medical knowing aware that most doctors themselves do not consciously articulate their reasoning in narrative terms although "storytelling" was assumed by many academics to be a natural human faculty (Bruner 1986), a point of contention that we consider in more depth later.

As noted above, early narrative medicine inevitably spreads its wings to embrace bioethics. What had traditionally been taken as a branch of moral philosophy focused on universal principles (paralleling an evidence-based approach) was revised through literary lenses. Where the specifics of the individual "case" had been absorbed into the general principles of beneficence, nonmaleficence, autonomy, and justice, Tod Chambers (1999) took these classic principles-based ethics cases and, drawing on literary theory, analysed them to expose their evident rhetoric. Chambers provocatively titled his 1999 text *The Fiction of Bioethics*, where he described bioethics cases not as factual accounts, but as inventive and persuasive narratives written by ethicists. Chambers' title implies that bioethics, claiming legitimacy as a rational, quasi-scientific enterprise, is in fact a form of story. Stated more pointedly, cases in the hands of principlists became analogous in literary terms to polemics that argue in favour of the espoused principles of their author.

According to Chambers, the various fictions themselves – as "case studies" – are of course not first-hand accounts of patients' experiences, but representations of those experiences. A later Hastings Center report, *Narrative Ethics: The Role of Stories in Bioethics*, edited by Martha Montello (2014), offered a roll call of key figures in narratively engaged bioethics at the time, such as Howard Brody, Rita Charon, Arthur Frank, Hilde Lindemann, and Anne Hudson Jones. These distinguished authors focused not only upon critical readings of representations of reciprocity and dialogue between patients and caregivers, but also advertised the use of established literary techniques such as close reading of ethics cases, as pioneered by Chambers.

A growing body of enthusiasts in medicine and healthcare eagerly took up narratology's ideas and techniques. This flowering was realised through innovative pedagogies such as viewing the patient-doctor relationship as one of co-construction of identity through an "agreed story" in "crafting relational identity" (Warmington 2020). Unfortunately for the field, an academic complacency set in, as reflected in a lack of self-critique and values clarification.

Now that we've just sketched the genesis of narrative in both general and medical contexts in North America, we turn to Eurocentric accounts. In a genealogical fashion, Jones and Tansey (2015) describe formal interest in narrative in medicine in the UK as originating from the early 1960s. This would trump the North American claim to priority in the field. British psychiatry had long employed story-based practices, psychoanalysis of course being dependent upon story. By focusing adult patients on memories of childhood, Freud also created temporal frames, forcing his patients into storying their symptoms; this narrativising was doubled in intensity as Freud wrote up his case studies with a narrative focus. (We should remember that Freud never won a Nobel Prize for science, where he was nominated multiple times. He did, however, win the Goethe Prize for Literature, celebrating his often exquisite case studies as literary storytelling.) In Freud's wake, many post-WWII British General Practitioners absorbed the seminal work of Michael Balint (1896–1970), a Hungarian psychoanalyst who spent most of his adult working life in England. His legacy is not just the ongoing existence of cathartic "Balint groups", but more so the larger reality sponsoring those groups: that medicine must acknowledge the importance of emotion and that the doctor-patient relationship is not just technical or instrumental, but potentially therapeutic on both sides. Drawing on Freud's and Balint's contributions, cracks begin to appear in contemporary narrative claims. Based on their work, although by no means restricted to them, we recognise that a major part of communication between patients and doctors is non-verbal and semiotic (signs and symbols) or, in an important sense, *pre*-narrative.

We focus on a particularly cogent summary involving narrative by Victoria Bates and Brian Hurwitz (2016), who point out that the establishment of what became known in the UK as "narrative-based medicine" was headlined by the 2015 decision of *The Lancet* to include narrative case studies rather than restrict reporting to purely instrumental accounts. Bates (a medical historian) and Hurwitz (a General Practitioner and medical historian) reach quite far back in time to offer an account of the roots of narrative in modern medicine, pointing to historical precedents in "the clinical casebooks of the early modern era" (ibid.: 559). Case reports in medicine, originally called "a narrative", can be traced to the 18th century and served two purposes. Individually, they afforded the singularity of illness, but collectively they offered diagnostic opportunity through classifications, such as typologies – "cancer cases", "heart cases", and later, following Freud, "studies of hysteria".

Interestingly, perhaps because they are historians first rather than scholars of literature, Bates and Hurwitz "use story and narrative almost interchangeably" (ibid.: 560), preferring the composite "history", which of course echoes the familiar patient history from medical practice. They point to etymological roots of both "history" and "story" that suggest commonalities (for example French *histoire*), then take a conceptual leap: "We take narrative to be the umbrella term for these *storia* and argue for their continuing valency in both medicine and 'the emergent discipline' of the medical humanities" (ibid.).

It is unclear, however, how the leap from *histoire* to narrative is made. Typically, in narrative medicine literature, a distinction is made between story and narrative, where patients offer "stories", while doctors and narrative medicine scholars make "narratives" out of these stories. Patients' "raw" stories are then "cooked" by medico-narrativists. Formally, "story" has been defined as the telling "of events unfolding in linear time", where a "narrative" is the formal "artful organization" of the raw materials of story "that may complicate their chronology, suggest their significance, emphasize their affect, or invite their interpretation" (Greene 2012). Conjoining "story" and "narrative", as Bates and Hurwitz do, avoids acknowledging the colonisation of "story" by the apparently more sophisticated, more professional sibling called "narrative." This would be impossible if the two were reconceived as one body, precluding the stalking, poaching, and colonising tendencies of the older sibling who assumes an air of sophistication.

One of the key concerns of contemporary narrative-based medicine returns us to the distinction often made between the patient's story and the medical narrative. Howard Brody (1994) in North America and John Launer (2002) in the UK were leading figures in making a case for a collaborative co-construction of narrative between patient and doctor. But this agreement on authentic story is complicated by the fact that although stories may be initiated in dyads, they are soon complicated by the development of rhizomatic relationships between carer, family, and health insurance networks, further complexified by artefactual and information webs. "Stories" are told and re-told such that plots multiply or overlap. Patients may be valorised as spiders at the centre of a web, but they can also be conceived of as a scattering of flies caught in the web, prey for the spider of medicine. In this way, supposedly "co-constructed" patient narratives become instead narratives of the occupier or imperialist. Theories, techniques, and schools of narrative medicine can occupy the same role of colonist, as we shall see. This is not an unexpected development, for the precedent was already well-established long before the narrative turn. Patients' stories, after all, are capital already claimed by medicine as they are re-formed and re-told in formal grand rounds, teaching occasions, published literature, informal talk amongst colleagues, and anecdotes shared with friends and acquaintances, despite ethical constraints. Such stories are even warmed over in disguised form as scripts in television medical soaps, where doctors are employed to advise on such scripts (Moody and Hallam 1998).

A brief note on illness narratives

The first book-length accounts of medical narratives that appeared in the second half of the 20th century are characterised as "illness narratives". For example, Arthur Kleinman (1988), in *The Illness Narratives*, called illness a disruption to biography that can prompt sense-making through reflection and writing, diaries being the common medium. Art Frank (1995), in his influential *The Wounded Storyteller*, concentrates on disruption of identity through illness, and the subsequent difficulties of articulating such a disjunctive self through writing. Jumping ahead to the present day, illness narratives now have critical mass, enough to constitute a genre: "autopathography". For example, Joanna Bourke (2014), in *The Story of*

Pain, stresses the use of a wide range of artefacts – such as diaries, letters, and poems – to articulate experiences of pain. Doctors too write about their suffering. The late neurosurgeon Paul Kalanithi's (2016) *When Breath Becomes Air* was completed by his wife after his death and became a best seller. Kalanithi died from lung cancer.

The cultural historian Thomas Lacquer (1989) claims that illness narratives afforded a new aesthetic genre, different from objective autopsy reports and case histories that introduced fictional and subjective elements, a precursor to contemporary "frontline" medical autobiographies and television soap operas, or "medical fictions" (Moody and Hallam 1998). Such narratives bounce back and forth between voices of patients and doctors. By the 1970s, these narrative forms were joined by ethnographers researching medical contexts, formally in terms of detailed linguistics (Byrne and Long 1976; Mishler 1985), and more informally as "dig where you stand" partial ethnographies sketching broad-brush accounts of medical life, including institutional contexts (Becker, Geer and Hughes 1961).

The imperialism of narrative: a variety of forms

In this section, we look at various ways in which narrative has morphed from a useful asset within the medical humanities large field of interest to a dominant form. Inevitably, with dominance comes oppression, and we show in the following chapters that time-based narrative-based medicine oppresses space-based lyric poetry. This matters because poetry is the art form par excellence for innovative metaphor production. Squash poetry and you deprive the medical humanities of a primary source of metaphor.

Naturalism morphs into imperialism

In large part because of Jerome Bruner's popularisation of narrative approaches to education and law, narrative became naturalised and then took a biological turn. For example, the highly respected historian Hayden White (1987: 1) says of narrative: "So natural is the impulse to narrate, so inevitable is the form of narrative for any report on the way things really happened, that narrativity could appear problematical only in a culture in which it was absent". In other words, narrative ways of thinking are habitual and normative; more, narrating is an "impulse" or a biological necessity. This claim rather complicates White's scenario of imagining "a culture in which it was absent". He cannot have it both ways: either narrativism is a biological imperative and then universal, or it is a cultural imperative and then takes on differing intensities and tones, with a possibility of absence. Further, and paradoxically for a biological impulse, narrative "report" is taken as a measure of veracity ("the way things really happened"). White then not only biologises but also scientises narrative. This makes narrative approaches more palatable for medicine.

Typical of the way that medicine and medical education have vigorously embraced the narrative wave is advertised in George Zaharias' uncritical (2018: 176) overview:

> Stories are our life's blood. We like to listen to stories, and it is through stories that we make sense of the world, that identity is shaped, and that we attempt to communicate what matters to us. … Narrative-based medicine (NBM) is the application of narrative ideas to the practice of medicine. Like patient-centred care, it came into being in reaction to the inadequacies of the biomedical model.

Taken from the perspective of "narrative-based medicine" itself, this is a fair summary of its claims. Read in a critical way, the passage makes inflated claims for narrative, along the way placing all narrative approaches under the one heading, while avoiding scrutiny and critique. What are the down-sides of narrative? Where does narrative hurt us? (As the remainder of this chapter will show, Zaharias' account is profoundly naïve.) Note the use of a biological metaphor, "life's blood", a rhetorical move that reads as reductively materialist and which echoes many other commentators' framing of narrativism as "natural". The inexorable destination of such arguments is towards the universality of narrative knowing. In time, "narrative" became a God-term, untouchable or immune to critique. This is what Jean-François Lyotard (1979) calls a "grand narrative", an overarching theme or method that can become ideological and oppressive.

Yet Lyotard too falls under the spell of story, as ideologies or Big Ideas are labelled "narratives", where the "local" or idiosyncratic "story" – such as a person's life history or patient's account of illness – becomes a "little narrative" or *petit récit*. As narrativism is applied to medicine, so doctors become interpellated in a particular ideological apparatus featuring the internalisation of a set of values that guide their actions. We grant that, if given only one choice to counter a biomedical scientism that peddles reduction and instrumentality, the narrativist ideology has some use. This, after all, was the rationale behind Rita Charon's (2001) original conception of a "parallel chart" as a qualitative counter to the standard (and necessarily reductive) quantitative clinical chart. However, if everyday narrative is indeed moulded by interpellation into Grand Narratives, then we must again look askance at Hayden White's claim that narrative recounting is total recall or "the way things really happened".

Charonian Narrative Medicine

The physician Rita Charon (Charon 2001, 2006; Charon and Montello 2002; Charon and Wyer 2008; Charon et al. 2016) and colleagues at Columbia University in New York make up the most high-profile group in narrative medicine. We capitalise this latter, more popular, variety as "Narrative Medicine". On occasion, we slyly and civilly question elements of Narrative Medicine by branding it as

Narrative Medicine™ to raise issues about what we see as a transformation of an educational enterprise into a business opportunity. This may be a particularly North American cultural feature. Charon (2001) initially formalised narrative ways of knowing as a parallel set of knowledge and skills to biomedical work, calling this "narrative competence" – an unfortunate choice of descriptor in a field where words matter. For us, "competence" is a weasel-word. It literally means "good enough", which we appreciate, yet it has become peacockish, signifying something more grandiose. If we stick to its root meaning, to be competent is to get over the line but not necessarily to show that extra zing that characterises capability, going beyond the necessary. Yet, we appreciate that for Charon (and many others in medical education) "competence" has come to connote a kind of supremacy, a mirror term to that other weasel-word "excellence".

Narrative Medicine's hard-earned capital is derived from investment in literary studies to better appreciate patients' stories – the raw matter from which the narratives are mined. Thus, Charon (Charon et al. 2016: 1) defines her version of narrative medicine as: "(a) rigorous intellectual and clinical discipline to fortify healthcare with the capacity to skilfully receive the accounts persons give of themselves – to recognize, absorb, interpret, and be moved to action by the stories of others". Despite the underlying promise of an innovative way of making a tender and caring relationship with a patient, we note that Narrative Medicine is couched in muscular, tough, hardtack talk: "rigorous", "discipline", "fortify", "capacity". The "discipline" allocates the empathy. Charon means business, both metaphorically and literally. There is then investment in tough-minded metaphors of Narrative Medicine's making and not from the patient's cache.

Charon (2016: 196) notes this distinction between the patient's story and the doctor's narrative in comments on "voice", relating to perspective or point of view: who is saying what and how might this be received and returned to the source? Victor Shklovsky, a Russian Formalist from the early 20th century discussed in more detail later, distinguished between *fabula* or what is described in an account (equivalent to the patient's story) and *syuzhet,* or how that original account is represented in text or talk (such as the case history). The mid-to-late 20th century French structuralists mirror this distinction in the terms *histoire* and *récit*, respectively, again a distinction glossed over by Victoria Bates and Brian Hurwitz discussed earlier, who collapse story and narrative into generic *histoire.*

Charon (2006: 40) defines "the major features of narrative" as: "Some event happens or state of affairs obtains within a temporal sequence and specified setting to and by characters or agents, and the opening state gives way to an altered state". (We note the awkward construction of this sentence and repetition of "state".) Further, she explains that a speaker somehow absorbs or represents the events from a particular point of view. The key elements for her are "time, characters, narrator, plot, and the relationships that obtain between teller and listener". We dispute none of this. Applying her defined narrative features to medicine, Charon (ibid.: 50) claims that plot is the *sine qua non* clinico-narrative intervention: "Clinical practice is consumed with emplotment. Diagnosis itself is the effort to impose a plot onto seemingly disconnected events or states of affairs". In our view, "[t]he effort to impose a plot" is clearly a directive even if it is done with understanding as its goal, and then a possible misdirection. "Effort" makes it muscular (again). It is not a revelation, an epiphany or sudden insight into the patient's condition, but rather an imposing of meaning along with a reconstruction. This doesn't seem to us to be a patient-centred diagnostic move, but at best an accurate and insightful apprehension of an essential truth of the patient's plight and/or of the encounter itself. But at the same time, it is inevitably a medicine-centred accruing of capital at the worker's (patient's) expense, as we have already explained. And at worse, we fear, it is a doctor-centred narrative oppression, a (possibly inadvertent, but nevertheless real) colonising of experience. The patient by now may have literally lost the plot, where it may have been appropriated by the doctor.

Lack of self-critique is apparent within the quasi-religious mission statement of Narrative Medicine™, where Charon (2016: 5) says: "All who seek care and all who seek to give care can unite in a clearing of safety, of purpose, of vision, of unconditional commitment to the interests of patients. This is the vision of narrative medicine". We are suspicious of both the piety and idealism of this vision statement, but there is a bigger problem. Throughout her work, advertised particularly in the single authored *Narrative Medicine: Honoring the Stories of Illness* (2006) and then in the multi-authored set of essays *The Principles and Practice of Narrative Medicine* (2016), there is – and by no means is this exclusive to Charon amongst the medical narrativists – an absence of reflexive self-critique. No sustained account of the model's limitations is extant. Although the 2016 text expands the scope of Narrative Medicine from the 2006 text in a welcome fashion (e.g., it has a greater emphasis on social justice and diversity), it still fails to critically address the epistemological assumptions of narrativism as applied to medicine and does not acknowledge (and answer) established critiques of narrativism generally, such as those of Galen Strawson and Angela Woods, discussed later. Such absence of self-critique extends to the failure to see how Narrative Medicine becomes complicit with biomedicine in a failed attempt at scientific legitimacy (Neilson 2022). This, rather than acting as translational device for a reductive biomedicine to aestheticise and politicise the latter.

Our next concern rests with the market monopolisation of the pedagogy of Narrative Medicine. Critical of the way that health insurance practices, backed by medicine, led to a dehumanising commodification, Narrative Medicine™ is now itself commodified, a business proposition based on the highly successful Master's programme at Columbia University, running since 2009; and in parallel workshops and seminars now run internationally. This is again why we continue to use the term Narrative Medicine™, fully aware that the weak cultural power of poetry prevents us from ever dreaming of such a lucrative product in our own field of interest. As Robert Graves said, "There is no money in poetry, but then there's no poetry in money, either" (one of our favourite critiques of bottom-line instrumentalism).

Where "[t]he goal of narrative medicine from its start has been to improve healthcare", surely this is no different from the aims of biomedicine where biomedical insight can lead to a correct diagnosis and treatment? Rather than projecting plot onto another's plot-less experience (is this any different than prescribing a pharmaceutical through biomedical diagnostics?), why not, again, take the given language of this experience (the patient's account) in its own right, as a *political* gesture? Consider Beckett's *Waiting for Godot* and how the sense of the thing is possible to plot, but also quite ridiculous. To understand this play, one must untether oneself from time and feel infinite dread in the face of the loss of a "storied" identity. Yes, the play unfolds in the time of performance, but what time is it in Purgatory, Mr. Wolf? Or, if we want to supplement the patient's account, why not politicise it in favour of that patient, acting as advocate for social justice? This is to take the lyric "I" of romantic poetry and turn it to the lyric "we" of socially aware, democratic poetry.

Rare critiques of narrativism's imperialism

Galen Strawson's huff

The catchphrase "It's the economy, stupid!" was coined by James Carville in 1992 while working on Bill Clinton's Presidential campaign team against George H.W. Bush. It is one of three such catch phrases the campaign brainstormed, but the only one that stuck. The unsuccessful other two were: "Change vs more of the same" and "Don't forget health care". Any decent rhetorician would have seen the last two as weak in comparison with the more memorable first. Of course, it's the "stupid" hook that is memorable. In contemporary medical education, we might say: "It's the narrative, stupid!" Oh, yes, of course! How stupid of me! The narrative imperative is insistent as we have seen and is largely resistant to critique. But some critics have put their heads above the parapet – most famously the British analytic philosopher Galen Strawson. In a review of Jerome Bruner's (2004) *Making Stories*, Strawson (2004b) sees an ouroboric worm at work, eating its own tail. Those who are already committed narrativists necessarily devour the idea that life and identity are storied, thus we get,

> On one side, the narrators: those who are indeed intensely narrative, self-storying, Homeric, in their sense of life and self, whether they look to the past or the future. On the other side, the non-narrators: those who live life in a fundamentally non-storytelling fashion, who may have little sense of, or interest in, their own history, nor any wish to give their life a certain narrative shape. In between lies the great continuum of mixed cases. How did the narrativist orthodoxy arise? I suspect that it is because those who write about it and treat it as a universal truth about the human condition tend, like Bruner, to be profoundly narrative types themselves.

We are not Strawson acolytes. We are sceptical about blunt typologies, or more, about pigeon-holing others. But we admire the fact that Strawson turns the tables on over-eager narratologists who claim that stories shape identity. For Strawson then, identity as a diachronic or "narrator" precedes the storying of life. Strawson's (2004a) critique of narrative orthodoxy (and then, by association, of narrative-based medicine) can be rejected as far too sweeping, even crude, but it remains sobering nevertheless. As a philosopher, he should recognise that his argument starts from an unproven premise with no confirmatory evidence: that there are "narrativists" and "non-narrativists" as explicit personality styles. Although Strawson recognises that these identities are on a spectrum, such typologies can be dangerous, hiding a range of subtleties and complexities. Strawson's sweeping critique has the paradoxical benefit of being refreshingly blunt however. He likes to poke in the eye: "At one point Bruner talks up the 'program in narrative medicine' recently instituted by Columbia University's College of Physicians and Surgeons, but all it amounts to is the idea that doctors should listen to their patients".

Recall again that the psychologist Bruner (1986) popularised the view of "Life as Narrative". Bruner's title holds open the possibility of other metaphors for life, yet he later argued that life *is* narrative, no longer a metaphor. Bruner concretised Hans Vaihinger's (1924) model of life as enactment of the philosophy of "as if", turning the speculative into the empirical "it is". Of course, "life as narrative" remains a metaphor, but a fossilised one, as harmful in its hegemony as "the body as machine" and "medicine as war". "Life is a story" is surely one metaphor amongst many.

Strawson (2004a) further argues – contra Bruner and others – that a narrative view of life is neither naturally given (the psychological view) nor naturally good (the ethical view), where not living in time is often seen as a form of madness. He distinguishes between a "diachronic" type who sees the world in narrative terms and assumes this is right and good; and an "episodic" type who does not perceive herself primarily as in a flow of time and does not see narrative perceptions as necessarily right or good, but may, for example, prefer spatial metaphors. Again, Strawson at least admits to "a great continuum of mixed cases", but if these exist then they confound rather than better articulate his typology. He takes Montaigne as an Ur-example of an episodic type who is uninterested in either recollection or what the future may hold, but lives in the (episodic) moment.

Strawson's intuitive argument offers no empirical evidence for its claims – they remain as provocations and suppositions. Despite claiming a "continuum of mixed cases", Strawson proceeds to set up an opposition between episodic and diachronic types as a rhetorical technique for engaging in conflict rather than conversation. Also, as Matti Hyvärinen (2012) notes, Strawson frames time in terms of a life history, but does not engage with the bigger world of time – human history, biological history as evolution, the planetary, or cosmic history as the consequence of the Big Bang. In anti-narrativism mode again, Strawson finds common ground with the poet Rainer Maria Rilke's remarks on the poetic imagination as a way of opposing "identity narrativism". Rilke says that the horizontally spreading lyric poem (as opposed to the vertical "story") is formed through intentional opposition to identity and ownership. The poet must uncouple from narrative identity, or storying oneself, by allowing the poem its own identity and liberty. It is through the poem that one achieves dissociation from a fixed identity while maintaining a sense of place. Only by dissolving the notion that the poem arises from "my" memory and is then "my" child do we give the poem the independence to roam and flourish, open to reception across a community of readership. In *Letters to a Young Poet*, Rilke (2013) says,

> Depict your sorrows and desires, your passing thoughts and beliefs in some kind of beauty – depict all that with heartfelt, quiet, humble sincerity and use to express yourself the things that surround you, … If your everyday life seems poor to you, do not accuse it; accuse yourself, tell yourself you are not poet enough to summon up its riches.

Here, Rilke expertly undoes subjectivity: know and "express yourself through the things that surround you". Poets closely notice such things, from which a self is sculpted. Perhaps the medicalised narrative overlaying the patient's story does not fit that story, but more, creates a sense of mistaken identity. In such cases, the patient, despite the best efforts of the narrative medicine-infused doctor, feels that she is "in" the doctor's story and not in hers. This is an old criticism of medical exchange dressed up in newer terms. The patient feels herself to be a misfit. A clear example of this is in practice comes with patients' resistance to prescriptions, crudely called "noncompliance" or "poor medication adherence" (Kleinsinger 2010).

Seamus O'Mahony, Angela Woods, and Crispin Sartwell enter the fray

By refusing to engage, narrative imperialism has so far survived external views critical of narrativity such as Seamus O'Mahony's (2013) work in medical education, when he speaks explicitly "against narrative medicine" as misreading of patients who do not present with "stories" but with disconnected pieces of information or fluctuating affect. In medical humanities, Angela Woods (2011a, 2011b) cautions against narrativism's overreach that suggests medical humanities enthusiasts haven't shown the courage to speak out against a dominant discourse of narrativism for fear of being side-lined. Woods writes with elegant scepticism towards narrative medicine and its over-reach, where "This has led to a neglect of other modes of reflecting upon and representing experience, such as poetry, phenomenological philosophy, or photography", all part of the broad spectrum of medical humanities (although Woods does not progress the case for these media). Woods provocatively asks if the search for meaning is a meta-narrative that we have every right to resist in the guise of narrative sceptics. She quotes the philosopher Crispin

Sartwell (2000), who says that in extremes, in ecstasy, in writhing pain, and of course in death, does narrative matter?

"Narratively speaking", suggests Sartwell, we are "not getting anywhere" in most of our trivial everyday activities. Yet in breathing, eating, watching television, walking around, and of course in sleeping, imagining, and dreaming, narrative time can be severely disrupted. Sartwell asks why we fail to take the apparently trivial non-narrative seriously. He asks also if we can take comfort in insignificance. Of course, as Woods points out, this is a message of discomfort that can also be taken as an inspiration. Is this not the point of an author such as Samuel Beckett who points to the absurdity of narrativity? Beckett's *Endgame* depicts the time-allergic act of becoming clogged, miring us in the certainty of uncertainty and the trivial instant:

> Moments for nothing, now as always, time was never and time is over, reckoning closed and story ended.

Let's release the grip of narrative

Alduy (undated) recognises that we need to "release the grip" of the narrative impulse, otherwise: "some of the most fundamental of human experiences … are stripped down from their intensity, beauty, horror, and maybe their truth, when we try to make sense of them by forcing them into a narrative box". Packing all literature into the narrative suitcase (as Narrative Medicine *in practice* appears to attempt) we squash important differences between genres and styles of writing that convey different meanings and address differing life events and experiences. There are then, says Alduy (ibid.):

> texts which defy, almost forbid, a purely narrative reading: poetic collections like those of Scève, Jaccottet, or Deguy, which create as much silence and white between the poems as to force other kinds of reading response and other metaphors to describe them (constellations, synchronicities, open ended repetitions that spiral in and out without coming back to center, even the "rhizome" dear to Guattari); picaresque novels or unfinished tales; fragments and elliptic aphorisms such as Pascal Quignard's; "grotesques" or "monstrous" essays as Montaigne describes them, where order is not a precondition for meaning...

We applaud Alduy's perceptive comment about creating "silence" and "white" in a text, as Beckett illustrates so powerfully (below). My goodness, how many times does "silence" appear in a clinical consultation as a key moment? These adventurous texts use narrative ironically, even parodically. Like poetry, Alduy suggests that such texts function as "devices crafted to open up new ways of thinking in multiple directions across or away from linear temporality". Narrative "force" – provided by plot structures that many see as story's main feature – may be missing in patients' presentations. This is in any case a kind of masculinising of narrative as per the "heroic venture" category in Propp's taxonomy of "tales" (discussed in the following chapter).

The problem with extending the boundaries of what constitutes "narrative" is that, eventually, almost anything goes. At this point, narrative becomes imperialistic by the back door – colonising literature simply by re-definition. For example, a patient's disconnected or incoherent account is narrative by default. Recall that one of Narrative Medicine's key functions is the superimposing of plot structures on patients' otherwise disconnected accounts. We find this a methodological paradox at the centre of narrative medicine: that consciousness is nonlinear, and yet narrative medicine seeks to emplot that which is plotless; or in Beckett's world, an animated suspension, or a palimpsest. We might amplify Beckett's deconstruction of narrative by drawing on Jacques Derrida's notion of "striking through" where narrative is permanently suspended, a "narrative-to-come" or a receding horizon. Beckett's "stories" occupy the space suspended narrative once occupied but has now vacated: narrative as vacant lot. You see, however, that no matter how much we try to park, transcend, or suspend narrative, it sticks like gum on the sole of the shoe.

Poetry need not do anything useful in medicine. We slyly suggest that a good start in appreciating its paradoxically useful uselessness in medicine is to separate it from the utility claims of narrative medicine. Beckett (1966) is again a good guide. In "Ping", a "short story" mentioned previously, he deconstructs the classic narrative account, and in the process offers us a poem-like thing:

All known all white bare white body fixed one yard legs joined like sewn. Light heat white floor one sure yard never seen. White walls one yard by two white ceiling one square yard never seen. Bare white body fixed only the eyes only just. Traces blurs light grey almost white on white. Hands hanging palms front white feet heels together right angle. Light heat white planes shining white bare white body fixed ping elsewhere.

"Ping" is just 908 words long, repeating phrases, such as "light heat white" and words, such as "traces". Striking out on a wholly associational, idiosyncratic direction here, we feel that "Ping" is as close as literature comes to orthopaedic surgery's "white out" arthroscopies. Time here is suspended. Beckett's room too is the white room of the clinic as imperium. Beckett brings the body to place in the descriptor, but then does something remarkable – he dissolves the body against the white of the background. It is an imperialism of white caught in its own box, but it is the opposite of colonising. The white spectre dissolves itself in its own substance. Deleuze and Guattari (2004b) call this a "de-territorialising" and dissolution of patrolled borders.

Beckett often claimed that his work meant nothing and was designed to signify nothing but failure. In *The Unnamable* (1953) he says: " … you must go on. I can't go on. I'll go on"; and in the story "Worstword Ho" (1983) that unpicks story from within, we are left with Beckett saying, equally famously: "Ever tried. Ever failed. No matter. Try again. Fail again. Fail better". So much for "narrative competence". What we have here is being, experience, and affect; a self-investment in meaning, a pouring of oneself into language's own performance. The result is not a steady decantation of insight or emplotment of a dot-to-dot in which point A leads to point B and the complete form of a patient and their illness picture is revealed; the result is an impression of movement from dot to dot, and a wonder at the movement itself.

Acknowledgement

This chapter was written in collaboration with Dr Shane Neilson.

10

ANOTHER TURN OF THE SCREW

As the good ship "poetry" leaves the harbour

Narrative medicine's roots in Russian Formalism

What are the roots of narrative studies? We opened the previous chapter with a tale of shifting terrain, as Peary tries to pinpoint the exact location of the North Pole where story (time) is collapsed into immediate space and place. Narrativism too was born on shifting terrain in the context of post-WWI revolutionary Russia, where one soon had to hold artistic ideas within the tight container of ideology. Russian Formalism started out as vaporising art for art's sake. But this view was soon denounced as bourgeois and the interpretation of texts became more strictly adherent to Marxist ideology. Terry Eagleton (1983: xi) places the beginnings of modern literary theory in 1917 with Victor Shklovsky's "pioneering essay 'Art as Device'". The title is a masterpiece of contradiction: art claims spearheads of innovation and yet is made functional. Art is engineered. To understand how narrative medicine has successfully bio-scientised, we must begin at the beginning, with Russian Formalism.

Russian Formalism invented the technique of "close reading" of literary texts – that analysis of a text can be done without any reference to external factors such as historical or cultural setting, purely from the nature of the text itself. Clinical medicine, in its reductive biomedical form, adopts a similar strategy where the patient is "read" purely for symptom expression so that a bodily based diagnosis can be made uncluttered by context such as the person's family or social life. We know, however, how myopic such a view can be: for example, a person living in a deprived social area has a shorter life expectancy than one living in a wealthy area. Sticking purely with the text is clearly limited to anyone with an anthropological, sociological, or political imagination for example.

DOI: 10.4324/9781003383260-11

Victor Shklovsky, "the self-proclaimed 'founder of the Russian School of Formal method'" (Steiner 1984: 44), had two major ideas: (1) a specific metaphorical orientation towards the accumulation and application of knowledge; and (2) the concept of "defamiliarisation" (*ostranenie*). Shklovsky defined the "Formal method" as "a return to craftsmanship" (ibid.: 45). His predominant metaphorical system for accumulating knowledge, as intimated in his definition, is a mechanistic one. As Steiner (ibid.) says, "Technology, that branch of knowledge pertaining to the art of human production, was the predominant metaphor applied by this model to the description and elucidation of artistic phenomena". We should note the parallels with medicine since Andreas Vesalius: medicine's key metaphoric system for structuring knowledge and guiding practice has been the "body as machine", where anatomy, and then medicine, is mechanics (Bleakley 2017: 55 passim). Shklovsky paradoxically wanted to break out of the very constraints he imposed through adopting an engineering metaphor for grappling with text through the process of defamiliarisation. Where medicine reads the patient as text (primarily a biomedical text), so the medical humanities afford a process of defamiliarisation that breaks out of the self-imposed habits of reductive biomedical readings to appreciate patients through a range of value systems: primarily, to repeat the mantra of this book, the aesthetic, ethical, and political. This radically intensifies and deepens the clinical encounter.

Steiner (1984: 45) relates some gossip from one of Shklovsky's colleagues, who called him a "fitter, a mechanic"; the case is made even more strongly with a comment made by Shklovsky to Roman Jakobson: "We know how life is made and how Don Quixote and the car are made too". Shklovsky's first method of close reading is one that reduces wholes into constituent parts, which is also how biomedicine reduces the human into tissue, and from there into cellular, molecular, and chemical components and processes. Shklovsky (in ibid.: 46) is refreshingly explicit about this:

> The understanding man scrutinizes the car serenely and comprehends 'what is for what': why it has so many cylinders and why it has big wheels, where its transmission is situated, and why its rear is cut in an acute angle and its radiator unpolished. This is the way one should read.

Following the Russian Formalists, let us extend metaphoric understanding to biomedical terrain in again scrutinising the engineering metaphors. Shklovsky (1991) is less interested in a somewhat Romantic sum of what is called "the human" when performing thought, but more in the specific neural connections firing at a specific moment in time: "In the theory of literature I am concerned with the study of the internal laws of literature. To draw a parallel with industry, I am interested neither in the situation in the world cotton market, nor in the policy of trusts, but only in the kinds of yarn and the methods of weaving". In other words, there is nothing of primary interest outside the matter of the text. Shklovsky's component part or constituent atom of literature was referred to as a "device", a creature of craft. The "device" itself is quite debatable as a useful, unique, and clear idea; in Eagleton's (1983: 3) summary: "sound, imagery, rhythm, syntax, metre, rhyme, narrative techniques, in fact the whole stock of formal literary elements".

So, does Shklovsky parallel biomedical reductionism in the sphere of literature as Rita Charon apparently does with her version of Narrative Medicine (Neilson 2022)? The answer is "no", because in parallel with this atomising Shklovsky intuited something truly important to understanding literature: defamiliarisation as a second core practice. So, while Shklovsky appears to crave reduction to instrumental values, where close reading of a text is like the inspection of a car engine, in fact this is just a prelude to the payoff gained from close inspection that is the twist in perception known as defamiliarisation – seeing familiar things anew. Defamiliarisation is the idea that *languages and practices used in art are deliberately artificial as a way of preventing the reader from processing a text or performance as information in an automatised, or perceptually habitual, way*. Put alternately, literature is language that calls attention to itself. More, returning to engineering, language must be tuned, and we must be attuned to it. Eagleton (1983: 3) expands:

> what distinguished [literary language] from other forms of discourse, was that it 'deformed' ordinary language in various ways ... by forcing us into a dramatic awareness of language, [literature] refreshes these habitual responses and renders objects more 'perceptible.' By having to grapple with language in a more strenuous, self-conscious way than usual, the world which that language contains is vividly renewed.

The primary way in which language is "deformed" is through metaphor use. To clarify this idea, the Formalists took further pains to distinguish between poetic and prosaic language. The difference was not in the presence or absence of symbols and imagery, for example, but rather that poetic language "was made artificially in such a way that perception lingers over it, thus reaching its greatest possible intensity and duration", whereas "[p]rose is normal speech: economical, easy, regular" (Steiner 1984: 147). Another Formalist, Jakubinski (in ibid.: 149), made a distinction quite useful for the current biomedical context:

> [l]inguistic phenomena ... should be classified, among other ways, from the standpoint of the goal for which the speaker exploits the verbal material in a given case. If he uses it for the purely practical goal of communication, we are dealing with the system of *practical language*, in which linguistic representations (sounds, morphemes, etc.) have no value in themselves but serve merely as a means of communication.

This is partly a misconception, as we have seen from previous chapters. Vernacular language is not necessarily prosaic but offers embodied metaphors (recall "panting for breath", or "vomiting blood"). Technical, reductive biomedical language in contrast is flat. But we know what the Formalists mean: poetry and creative prose are an exception to everyday speech, where the metaphor count in the former is purposefully high and innovative such that language transcends mere communication. Jakubinski (ibid.) continues, "Other linguistic systems are conceivable (and exist) in which the practical goal retreats into the background and linguistic combinations acquire a value in themselves. ... I conditionally call this system verse language". Further:

> In practical language the semantic aspect of the word (its meaning) is more prominent than its sound aspect ... details of pronunciation reach our consciousness only if they serve to differentiate the meaning of words .... Thus various considerations compel us to recognize that in *practical language sounds do not attract our attention*. It is the other way around in verse language. There, one can claim that sounds enter the bright field of consciousness and attract our attention.
>
> *(ibid.: 149, 150)*

If anyone reading this has attended a Narrative Medicine seminar and been taught "narrative competence", then your alarm bells should be going off, for what you're really being taught is Russian Formalism to both improve your practice and, supposedly, to also revivify your working soul. Charon's mini history of close reading misses its origin point with the Russian Formalists in 1917 where she begins with I.A. Richards, a British scholar active in the 1920s and the poet and critic William Empson's tutor at the University of Cambridge. We find this odd, for what Charon (2016: 166) has been vending since her movement started sounds a lot like Shklovsky's promise:

> [r]igorous training in close reading – at least narrative medicine's version of close reading – improves readers' capacity for attention but also revolutionizes the reader's position in life from being an onlooker checking the log of past events to becoming a daring participant in the emergence of reality.

Again, grandiose claims, inflated language: not just engaging in life, but "daring" and emerging from the fog of misunderstanding to face "the emergence of reality". Just like Shklovsky famously wanted to reveal, through poetry, the "stoniness of the stone", so Charon wants to make the patient "patiently" again. But does it matter that Charon's origin myth for close reading is Richards rather than Shklovsky? We think so, in terms of subtlety of technique, where Russian Formalism's kind of close reading is more "molecular", to use Nikolas Rose's (2007: 3, 11) terminology, where: "biomedicine visualizes life at ... the molecular level", which "is itself enmeshed in a 'molecular' style of thought about life itself". To draw on the phenomenon of fractals, where patterns are repeated at differing magnitudes, we see Shklovsky's critical molecular eye as one that captures wholeness and complexity at the level of small detail. Rose is right to recognise that just as close reading need not be reductive, so biomedicine need not be reductive. Rather, it can be granular but encompassing. Complexity occurs at different levels of organisation.

The appeal of Russian Formalism for Narrative Medicine seems natural, for the Formalists were very much invested in transforming the study of literature into a science of qualities (Nielson 2022), while Narrative Medicine has gradually adopted a practical orientation to prove itself in the image of Evidence-Based Medicine (as "Narrative Evidence Based Medicine") (Charon and Wyer 2008). Jakobson (in ibid.: 23) referred to what we would now call "literary studies" as a "science", whose objective was extracting (and abstracting) an essence: "The object of literary science is not literature but literariness, i.e., what makes a given work a literary work". Eichenbaum (in ibid.: 22), a member of the St. Petersburg-based Society for the Study of Poetic Language and a colleague of Shklovsky's, wrote:

the Formal method, by gradually evolving and extending its field of inquiry, has completely exceeded what was traditionally called methodology and is turning into a special science that treats literature as a specific series of facts... What characterizes us is neither 'Formalism' as an aesthetic theory, nor 'methodology' as a closed scientific system, but only the striving to establish, on the basis of specific properties of the literary material, an independent literary science.

In their enterprise to taxonomise language, the Russian Formalists reduced language to its constituent parts, again conceiving of it in mechanistic terms through engineering metaphors, so that the enterprise itself could be called a science, as a legitimising strategy: "What is significant about the Formal method?" Shklovsky wrote in his characteristic staccato style:

What is significant is that we approached art as production. Spoke of it alone. Viewed it not as a reflection. Found the specific features of the genus. Began to establish the basic tendencies of form. Grasped that on a large scale there is a real homogeneity in the laws informing works. Hence, the science [of literature] is possible.

(in ibid.: 65)

Here, surely, is a logic for Narrative Medicine's desire for scientific legitimacy that it has overlooked: a striking similarity between biomedicine and Russian Formalism. For Shklovsky, the Formal method not only reduces language to its constituent parts and taxonomises, but also discovers "basic tendencies of form" and demonstrates that there "is a real homogeneity in the laws informing works". It is the latter qualities that Shklovsky quite rightly identifies as the hallmarks of Western science. Shklovsky seems to describe what we would now think of as fractals within complexity science – that the same form can repeat itself at differing magnitudes.

Where Russian Formalism and Narrative Medicine part company is in the former's rebellious embrace of art for art's sake, refusing to consider that art affords a reflection of, for example, a sociology or psychology of the conditions that produced it. As Shklovsky maintained in what has been called "arguably one of the best known paragraphs in aesthetic history": "In order to restore our lived experience of the world and feel things again, in order to make a stone a stone again, we have something called art" (in Yakubinski 2018: 16).

Shklovsky's point is transparent – he configured literature and criticism as science but was not interested in turning science into literary forms. But, following the theme of this book, science can indeed be raised from its instrumental slumbers to sing – by embracing other value positions. The register of science can be raised from instrumental quantitative to aesthetic qualitative, introducing beauty, morality, and justice for example. Russian Formalism was both an instrument of interpretation and of amplification: deepening and intensifying qualities. We offer the scientific theme and aspiration of the Formalists as a unique connection, with the caveat that the Formalists were part of the same cultural milieu inspired by the philosophy of positivism. Here, "only scientifically verifiable propositions" have meaning (Goldenberg 2006: 2622). Steiner (1984: 253), the definitive historian of the Russian Formalists, suggests that positivism circulating as far back as the 1870s was an influence. The Formalists and biomedicalists adopt the political stance that art and medical science are both decontextualised, depoliticised, valueless enterprises (or rather they generate their own value from a base of functionalism), yet this is reflective of a larger cultural turn that cannot be isolated as egregiously abnormal or unique.

Problems of definition: narrative as Procrustes' bed

Let us return to principles. As raised earlier, an interesting question for us is: What kinds of stories are legitimate in the Narrative Medicine purview? For example, Samuel Beckett's prose poem *Ping* (http://remue.net/IMG/pdf/Ping.pdf), an excerpt of which closed the previous chapter, is worth a reprise. *Ping* defies classification. It is a prose piece refusing explicit narrative elements, aspiring to the formal mathematical symmetry of some conceptual poetry while not blanching out affect (it raises a productive chill in us):

> All known all white bare white body fixed one yard legs joined like sewn. Light heat white floor one square yard never seen. White walls one yard by two white ceiling one square yard never seen. Bare white body fixed only the eyes only just. Traces blurs light grey almost white on white. Hands hanging palms front white feet heels together right angle. …

So, if patients tell stories and doctors convert them to narratives; or, if patients and doctors co-construct stories, is there anybody out there in narrative medicine who is drawing lines between "stories" and jibberish? And does this matter? Beckett doesn't write jibberish – his stories/poems are carefully constructed uses of language. The character is (literally as well as figuratively) suspended, made into a ghost, and absorbed into the background ("never seen", "only just", "traces", "blurs", "almost white", "white on white"). Isn't this how we feel when desperately ill? The story is a whiteout but not a whitewash. Beckett subverts the whole notion of plot as an ironic gesture; and his characters are similarly disembodied embodiments (actually, Beckett is smarter than this game-playing). We suggest in any case that spatiality-sensitive and image-based lyric poetry is a better medium of appreciation and critical awareness with which to approach Beckett than classic narratology. But we are at a loss to say where a "story" disintegrates or represents a mind in turmoil for example.

Is a postmodern deconstruction of "story" (purposefully not developing character or plot for example) still a story? Is story the same as tale, and is tale different from anecdote? As noted in the previous chapter, Vladimir Propp's (1968) classic analysis of folk tales in the Russian Formalist tradition reveals 31 dimensions. Move outward from the classic folk tale to other story genres and, as Cecile Alduy (undated) suggests, "the word 'narrative' requires some elucidation", so that for narrative-based medicine,

> what we really mean is a certain kind of narrative: not the picaresque, not the Joycean (in other words, neither the early nor the postmodern), but the good old Aristotelian (reincarnated nowadays in the Hollywood template, or even, the makeover reality show success stories, which by the way, fall perfectly into Propp's morphology of the folk tale, complete with opponents, obstacles).

Retreating then to Propp's morphology as a framework for narrative understanding and appreciation would be a little like relying entirely on classical anatomy to practice medicine – a rusting, reductive framework that by-passes anti-narrativists who write stories, such as Beckett above, Clarice Lispector, Lydia Davis, Thomas Pynchon, David Foster Wallace, Angela Carter, Gil Orlovitz, William Gaddis, and so forth. These writers revel in paratext, subtext, intertext, dissolved text, but not in classical "story". So, when we see the banner "narrative-based medicine" we can safely assume that "story" refers only to the classic arc of the plot and to characters with substance and not Beckett's ghost. But what kinds of stories are told, and what kinds of characters do the telling, in bodily and mental distress?

Robert Centor (2007) keeps the narrative faith where he suggests that,

> … the great physicians differ from the good physicians because they understand the entire story. Only when we understand the complete story do we make consistent diagnoses. Each patient represents a story. That story includes their diseases, their new problem, their social situation, and their beliefs. How do we understand the story? We must develop excellent communication skills and gather the history in appropriate depth. We must perform a targeted physical

examination based on the historical clues. We must order the correct diagnostic tests, and interpret them in the context of the history and physical exam. Once we collect the appropriate data, we then should construct that patient's story. The story includes making the correct diagnosis or diagnoses. The story must describe the patient's context. … Understand the full story.

Feel free to make a drinking game with the appearance of the word "story"! A physician, John (2013: 57), makes a plea for a shift from doctor-centred to patient-centred practice, drawing on another of Osler's maxims that runs: "it is much more important to know what sort of patient has a disease than what sort of disease a patient has". And John goes on to say: "The patient should always be allowed to describe his symptoms and sensations using his own words". So far, so patient-centred. This, says John, is the patient's "story". But inevitably:

The doctor then duly moves on to closed questions, which are used to confirm specifics and understand the cause of symptoms in a more technical context. Indeed, as the consultation progresses closed questions can be used successfully to focus specific areas that maybe do not emerge from the patient's *story* during the initial open-question session.

Two issues emerge from this: first, again, is the patient necessarily telling a story in recounting disconnected issues, facts, and feelings every time she speaks? And second, what will the tactics of representation be and how will the patient's labour be rewarded and honoured? The ball in John's account again falls into the hands of the doctor.

Rita Charon (2006: 99) wants it both ways, where: "[u]sually, the story of sickness comes out chaotically, achronologically", and then proceeds to recommend imposing "plot" to restore chronology. But is this move – one of decreasing uncertainty – for the sake of the patient or the physician? There can be achronological stories. But where does imposition of plot end? In the service of diagnosis, such an imposition may seem justified, but this appears to compromise authentic patient-centredness as reflected in co-construction of meanings between doctors and patients. Practically speaking, making sense of things is important. But what are the limitations to emplotment? And when does emplotment just not apply? We suspect the imposition is vast. We are nervous about claims for patient-centredness that are doctor-centred emplotments. Stories are returned to patients with interest say the medico-narrativists, but such "returning" surely remains doctor-centred even if the intentions are good. Indeed, there are echoes here of colonialism, albeit well-intentioned.

Hans Duvefelt (2016) is also wary of "storying" medical encounters as literalising:

Sir William Osler wasn't exactly wrong when he said, "Listen to your patient, he is telling you the diagnosis." But he didn't mean it literally. His patients did not offer up esoteric and complete medical diagnoses on a silver platter. They left him clues in plain language that he listened to carefully in order to make the correct diagnosis. He penned his words in an era when medical information was scarce among non-medical people. There was no Dr. Google, Dr. Oz or Dr. House to educate the public about diseases or medical terminology a century ago.

An apocryphal story from the same author (in the age of Dr Google) also shows that when stories are told, they may be unhelpful in reaching a diagnosis:

> Mrs. LaVerdiere made an appointment for nausea some time ago. As soon as I walked into the exam room, she started telling me about how she must have eaten a spoiled crab sandwich on her trip to a coastal fishing village the weekend before. Her conversation was full of theories as to why she was feeling unwell and her husband wasn't. I finally got her to describe in great detail exactly what she felt, and the gnawing pain that radiated to her back did not fit with a simple case of food poisoning. Her CT scan showed the smallest pancreatic cancer ever diagnosed at Cityside Hospital, and she underwent a Whipple procedure as easily as any routine minor surgery.
>
> *(ibid.)*

As an aside on the veracity of the account, Whipple procedures are known to leave patients very ill, something Duvefelt omits. However, the procedure may be the only chance a patient has of a cure. Further, patients sometimes do not tell *their* stories faithfully, but rather recount incidents in a lay "medicalese" that they think will suit their doctor's mindset:

> Mrs. Waller describes ordinary bodily sensations in the most dramatic terms and throws terminology around that rocks me out of my country-doctor way of plain-talking. She has, over the years, described ordinary itches as "you know how it feels when you've been bitten by a thousand fire ants," headaches as "I felt like I was about to pop a berry aneurysm" and indigestion as "pyloric stricture." I have the distinct impression she is always trying to make my job easier by describing things in more or less medical terms in case I forgot to speak English.

In an analysis that describes the three main ways in which patients' stories can be confounded, Duvefelt (ibid.) explores the above example of talking in medicalese – often picked up from the Internet – as if this will please the doctor. Such acquired patient-speak thus offers theories and diagnoses rather than plainly describing symptoms. This can frustrate doctors. As for the other ways, some people are simply unable to recognise what they are feeling (as sensations), or to adequately describe emotions. Instead, they report what other people observe of their behaviour. In this way, they are strange collateral historians of themselves. The final way comes when bodily sensations are described rather than the emotions that accompany them, such as anxiety. In this case, we have a so-called "physical" focus with emotions either un-narrated or, as is more often the case, shunted onto a physical target. We do not find in Narrative Medicine's version of close reading adequate ways to deal with these sublimated and sideways narratives.

We do not know the answer to this because nobody has done the empirical research, but we might ask: (i) what are the innovative metaphor yields of patient talk as opposed to doctor talk within the consultation; and (ii) is higher innovative metaphor yield positively correlated with both diagnostic accuracy and patient recovery? To this issue of diagnostic accuracy and best treatment or care, we might add that in psychiatry it is obvious to all that the way a patient tells a story is filtered through presenting psychological conditions – thus a person labelled as hysteric tells a story flamboyantly; an anxious person stutters and fumbles her way through an account; a depressed person relates a story as if under a thundercloud; a paranoid person tells a story larded with suspicion or unjustified accusation; a person labelled as psychotic offers either a mass of bizarre and disconnected detail to the normative hearer, or a meticulous and detailed factual account with no colour, nor an ounce of feeling. These examples are given non-judgementally and of course are open to objection as generalisations and even stereotypes. Here, *the manner of telling a "story" is probably more important or revealing than the story itself.* We are not convinced that Narrative Medicine adequately addresses this question of tone or style.

And so, to poetry: key ideas for a lyrical medicine

In summary of our concerns, and accepting that in Charon and colleagues' 2016 text, some authors do tackle a couple of more complex narratives (for example, Spiegel and Spencer take on Alison Bechdel's graphic memoir), we are left with one thought: who is taking on space- and place-based, atemporal lyric poetry in the Narrative Medicine camp? Irvine and Charon (2016: 113) mention, through a quote from Cleanth Brooks, a literary theorist, that poetry "cannot be paraphrased" but then compare such a poetry-sensitive insight with their concept of story: "In a like manner, a story is something whose content cannot be reduced to analyzable data". Well, if the patient tells the story and the doctor creates the plotmarks and the narrative forms, and then hands this back to the patient as an accurate diagnosis, but offered with a caring attitude, that in turn demands a biomedically based intervention from the thousands available – say a course of antibiotics – how exactly is this not paraphrasing and reducing the story to analysable data?

Abraham Verghese (in Dolan 2015), even as a narrative enthusiast, recognises that patients' "histories" as stories may have no resolution, epiphany, or significant use of dramatic forms. They may be flat as they are told, or so supremely convoluted as to shake off "plot" (ask psychiatrists who have treated both the deeply depressed and the deluded). Further, the quality of the doctor-patient relationship is primarily achieved through the character and capability of the doctor's performance in the physical examination, using hands-on examination focused on here-and-now acute use of the senses, or what Verghese calls "the animal snout". Here, *topos* trumps *tempus*. Musicality and sound are prior to prose but not poetry, which is sound.

Verghese (2015) suggests that frustrating the patient's story may be a problem of medicine's own making: first as habitual rapid intervention, where the doctor typically interrupts 11 seconds into the consultation (Ospina et al. 2018); and second as the engineered exchange of the physical examination to remote imaging (with the understanding that such testing is preferable because of its accuracy, one of biomedicine's supposed gifts. But what test is truly accurate if not informed by a whole clinical picture?). In particular, and unconsciously beckoning poetry, Verghese bemoans the lack of inventiveness in coining new medical metaphors – as we note throughout – thus falling back habitually on tired examples. This leads to "an atrophy of our imagination" (ibid.: 232, 233). Here, we suggest that narrative medicine suffers from the symptom of "thick slicing", or lack of discrimination. This is the opposite of "thick description" that narrative medicine borrows from anthropology (Clifford Geertz in particular) (Geertz 1973), where the patient's "thin" story is given body through narratalogical interventions and re-readings (Charon et al. 2016: 22). In contrast, Verghese (2015: 234) warns against purloining the patient's story in the name of medicine, where "the voice of medicine" must not be mistaken for the "voice of the patient". The inherent problem is: who is in control of the narrative? It is still the doctors who have learned and applied narrative medicine, despite their claims for co-construction of story with patients.

The anatomy of the clinical encounter is not comprised just of talk, yet imperial narrativism privileges the lexical, largely ignores sonics, the non-verbal (proxemics, gestures, tics, eye contact, touch, movement, paralinguistics) and semiotic. A range of gestures, intonations, silences, and accompanying signs and symbols largely fail to register in narrative medicine accounts. Maura Spiegel and Danielle Spencer (in Charon et al. 2016: 23), in the context of Narrative Medicine's "narrative competence", do note that understanding and reading patients' nonverbal gestures is important to intersubjectivity, where: "In the clinical encounter … gestures, facial expressions, and body language can signal in such significant ways". Further, the authors also note how nonverbal communications can both support and contradict the verbal and can be ambiguous and are singularly contextualised.

But their account of the nonverbal is not adequate – we want to know about the rhythm and musicality of encounters; about lifting off the beat; about syncopation and silences; and about preverbal utterances, grunts, and groans of pleasure. It took a graphic narrative for Charon and colleagues to insert the nonverbal into their narratology frame, which seems a little cheap. They could have learned so much from gapping words in the field à la Charles Olson, Anne Carson's experimental forms, blocking words into concrete forms like Beckett, or exquisite, stripped phrasing from Louise Glück that leaves no tree unpruned. This, after all, is the vernacular – the way that we speak, especially in the pressing context of an emotionally stirred patient trying to describe symptom: sometimes sticking and stumbling over words, sometimes stunned into silence, and at other times eloquent and on point.

A patient recounting her own history of symptom may work backwards, unravelling plotlines rather than developing plots: the patient's "story" "un-storying" like an ouroboric snake eating itself from the tail. Indeed, words may be secondary here to the musicality of utterances: symptom expressed as the "blues", emphasis on atonality, an opening up of the sonic spaces into which words wander but have nothing to say: stunned into silence by circulating pains, discomforts, sickness. Semiotics-in-action is often a world of sticky signs that act like flypapers. As both patient and doctor utter words, so they stick to the flypaper that is "the consultation"; but such utterances may be dead upon arrival. Our point being that a clinical encounter affords unpredictably in passage and may mess with conventional notions of "storied" encounters.

The 18th-century Viennese physician Leopold Auenbrugger, who first identified the potential for percussion of the body, was a keen musician who once invited Mozart to play at his home (Bleakley 2020b). Auenbrugger saw the potential for diagnoses not just in physical examination but also in lung and breath sounds such as crackles or alveolar rales. Our point is that patients' rational "talk" is co-extensive with the unpredictable musicality of primal, preverbal somatic interruptions, where illogical gargling, filler words, and grunts may upset what was up to now a perfectly lucid account. Such preverbal and nonverbal elements "thicken" the story, and we need expertise in translation to read them. The way this is being theorised is akin to semiotics – signs and symbols in context, to include the world of objects and their significance in the clinical encounter. We say "akin" because, in our view, nonverbal communication is not recognised as independent referents with a spatial and sonic character but rather intrinsically as part of the "narrative" in Narrative Medicine. All is sucked into analysable utterance. Yet poetic/spatial awareness of the nonverbal is standard fare for the psychotherapist, clinical psychologist, and psychiatrist, so Narrative Medicine's narrative competences may not be the best stop from which to alight from the bus for learning such thick description capabilities where they are thick sliced.

Doctors are semioticians before they are narrativists, users of signs and symbols grounded in pathophysiology, and prompting for clearer information about symptom expression through formulaic means such as oppositional categories or semantic qualifiers (such as "is it a sharp or a dull pain?" "Does it hurt all the time or only at certain times?"). The patient will have a "front story" that is their discussion with the doctor, and a "back story" that is just as important and is not revealed. The backstory is probably laden with affect that is central to the patient's care needs. The backstory is then no story at all, but a spatially sensitive constellation of half-explored and semi-articulated affect. Psychoanalysts will say that this unconscious backstory is shaping the encounter – but is it a back*story*, or a back*space*? We suspect it is both, a locker brewing metaphors and a storeroom of prescribed metonyms.

Enter poetry, by the back door. Where narrative medicine models Procrustes' bed, utterances are then stretched to fit a preconceived notion, missing the extra-narrative intentions of lyrical verse. Let us give an illustrative example. We critique Schleifer and Vannatta's (2013: 181–3) analysis of William Carlos Williams' poem "The Red Wheelbarrow", occurring as it does within the Narrative Medicine frame. We do this not to belabour our already-established critique of Narrative Medicine itself, although indeed our criticisms that follow track back to that critique. Instead, we carefully walk through this narrativisation of "The Red Wheelbarrow" as the very field from which the case for a lyrical medicine can be made. Our concern is that the poem is not read as poem but is (unnecessarily in our view) treated as prose and then subjected to narrative forces. In other words, poetry is forced into the narrative mould. Williams' poem runs:

so much depends
upon

a red wheel
barrow

glazed with rain
water

beside the white
chickens

Here, say the authors, "a significant feature of 'The Red Wheelbarrow' is that it implies some kind of narrative, a story with a beginning, middle, and end". As poets, we disagree. "Implies" is key here – lots of stuff can imply a narrative where the story is projected on to an event as an afterthought. What is captured here is a suspended moment in time: not just the event described in the poem, one comprising images (rain, chicken, wheelbarrow), but also the framing meta-reflection ("so much depends") upon *these* objects, at *this* time.

The poem suggests something immense in a minimalist space (precisely what Minimalism promises), and it is the nature of the images and their connection that is this poem's meaning, if it could be called that. There is no narrative here except whatever plot is imposed upon it. The speaker is undefined. There is no conflict. There is only an eternity, and this instantiation of Narrative Medicine has no apparatus to appreciate it. But the event itself may be best described poetically, as Williams does in the original text. We don't deride this narrativistic impulse, for it is speculative, and we salute the speculative. What we abhor is what is ubiquitous in the field: a resort to default (narrative) in the absence of the capacity or ability to analyse the poetry (as poetry).

Also, let's not interfere with the artistic credibility of the poet who wants to *show* and not necessarily *imply*. We described the phenomenological moment that so intrigued Husserl, of the object showing itself. Poems also thrive on implication of course, but primarily they show or reveal, and in close-up as *ekphrasis* or close noticing. We note this as an ecological perception, a two-way process: the object displays as we display the object in words. Schleifer and Vannatta (ibid.), however, drawing on the detective genre, turn Williams' raw statements into a guessing game, a puzzle to be solved. They begin by stitching the consciously structured poem into one continuous line: "so much depends upon a red wheelbarrow glazed with rainwater beside the white chickens". Now this makes no sense as story and most importantly Williams didn't compose an uninterrupted line. What it does reveal is a preference on the part of the authors for the narrative form. Indeed, running the poem's lines together ruins both the rhythm and startling imagery of the poem *as poem*.

There is mystery afoot perhaps ("so much depends") but the "characters" (wheelbarrow, rainwater, chickens) are undeveloped – even if the wheelbarrow is a striking red, more so because of the rainwater glaze – and there is no evidence of plot. Indeed, the strikingly plain representation of the objects is the very poetic diction that makes this a brilliant Minimalist poem. The objects are simply there, radiant in their uncomplicated presence, one beside another. In other words, they are *placed*. Getting placed in space is, suggests the philosopher Ed Casey (2013), the primary phenomenological gesture – it is the very appearance of the object. To say that the objects are the narrative (along with the metareflection "so much depends") is like calling the ocean floor a desert.

Yet Williams does poetically complicate the issue by three main devices of implication and explication. First, the opening stanza of implication sets a mystery. Just what depends upon the wheelbarrow and chicken: the farmer's livelihood, or the self-worth of the wheelbarrow and the chickens in their own right? Further, Williams does not say: "much depends" but injects suspense, as "so much depends". The second device is one of explication – enjambment (from the French *enjambement* "to stride over", "to go beyond"). This is a much-used technique where a line is not punctuated but falls or slides away into the following line with a sudden surprise. So, "so much depends upon" is mild in comparison with the sudden step "so much depends/upon", making us eager to find out what the "so much" refers to. Again, running the poem into a single line obliterates the enjambment, ignoring a key structural device.

Third, and explicit, the poem is entirely removed from temporal reference. "So much depends" can be read as a reference to the future, but the poem is anchored in the instantaneity of the event, the bringing together of rainwater, glazing and wheelbarrow standing beside chickens grounded in space. Hence, the poem is purposefully structured through poetic diction as lyric poem and not as continuous narrative arc. We will now consider the poem as (gasp) a poem! – an ambiguous thing that need not be tamed, for production of ambiguity is the birth-right of the artist, and what is feared in diagnostic medicine.

In what sense does our quite lengthy exegesis of Williams' poem help with medical work or medical education? Such poems do have medical implications, not just because Williams was a doctor, but also because this is an exercise in close noticing and witnessing, capabilities essential to the clinical encounter. We are completely on board with Rita Charon's teachings in this regard. You might see Williams' poem as presenting a slim noticing, stripped back to fundamentals. But isn't this precisely what medical students are taught to do, to boil down excess to dry essences as the hard tack of the diagnosis? We thereby highlight the special quality of Williams' work, in which a minimalist style seems to mimic the flattening quality of the biomedical epistemology, and yet analysing it as poetry seems to reclaim its richness, a richness that, in truth, was ineradicable. This is a paradox at the heart of the methodology of what we call "Lyrical Medicine" (Bleakley and Neilson 2021), a key component of the medical humanities.

To be fair, Schleifer and Vannatta (2013: 181, 182) note that Williams' "The Red Wheelbarrow" "observes details in the environment and asserts value". But they simultaneously denature the poem by forcing it to take on the identity of narrative, admitting themselves from the start that this is perhaps a mistaken reading: "even when a poem does not present an explicit narrative, as in Dr. William Carlos Williams' famous poem 'The Red Wheelbarrow', it can help us learn to recognize and recover narrative knowledge". This seems like pretty slim pickings for narrative enthusiasts and, again, misses the poem *as poem*; in so doing, it abuses the work.

The rationale is that patients do not present whole narratives but bits of story that must be pieced together. So, Williams' poem is taken as an example of fragmentary evidence of a wider story and is narrativised as exercise. Well, yes. The observations Williams makes are necessarily embedded in a wider scene, but again the whole point of making the poem may be to offer the frozen scene as exquisitely beautiful and right, as complete. What is the point in doing the wrong exercises? Do we go to the gym to lift weights but somehow end up swimming instead? Williams offers a kind of moral about suspending interference. Time is explicitly suspended for a reason, so that things can show themselves. As we will insist, poets often like to dig where they stand.

Schleifer and Vannatta (ibid.) continue: "The story presents itself as a series of disparate facts, emotions, anecdotes" where "these elements of narrative and significance need to be gathered together to make a meaningful whole". Well, no: these are not "elements of narrative". What facts other than the possible physical fact of represented objects? We contend that there is not a single emotion named in the poem, and if there is an anecdote, we're at a loss. Signs of resting are projected on to a poem that stands outside the limits of "story". But they are certainly "elements of ... significance". The authors then assert: "practice and training in the interpretation of poetry is particularly useful in developing the competence of health care workers in recovering the information and meaning of a patient's story". Though we appreciate the advocacy for poetry in this instance, we point out that the authors are in a sticky position. Not only do they force poetry into the narrative box, but they also compound the problem by resorting to instrumentalism.

Ultimately, after an understanding has been cultivated such that poems are appreciated as poems, then we cautiously endorse the application of this knowledge to clinical encounters. This is lyrical medicine. But skipping straight to the applied mode has wreaked such havoc in the medical and health humanities. What if healthcare workers were introduced to poetry as a strangeness they never knew they needed, for their own selves; that they should cultivate their own relationship with poetry in order to cultivate their own relationship with themselves? What if selfhood were made strange, leading to defamiliarisation? What if a space were created between poetry and its application, again a plot that can be cultivated as field? What might happen then?

Schleifer and Vannatta freely admit that poetry helps us to deepen experience of phenomena, recognising that Williams' opening line "so much depends" orients us to value, rather than to information as objective fact. They derive a metaphor of their own, that Williams is telling us that the everyday is "glazed with value". Finally, a poetic insight, an epiphany! Such appreciation of poetry can alert us to the manner of presentation of patients and not just, in Schleifer's and Vannatta's words, "presented *information*" (italics in original), undermining their previous advice to recover the "information" of a patient's "story".

From our experience, often it is not the conversation between doctor and patient or psychotherapist and client that matters, but the space that has opened in the place where differing foci fail to meet or only partially meet. Discontinuity and surprise regularly inhabit the accounts of patients consulting with doctors and clients with psychotherapists. Sometimes this adds up to a mistranslation. When patients describe symptoms – and events surrounding symptom appearance and development – are they, as the celebrated late 19th-century doctor and medical educator William Osler hints, telling stories ("Listen to your patient; he is telling you the diagnosis")? We say "hints" because Osler does not actually say "listen to your patient's *story*" but rather just "listen to your patient, he is telling you the diagnosis".

Medicine and medical education need not necessarily be sucked into the vortex of narrative, but can represent poetry's engagement with things, which is poetry's forte: bringing the objects of the world into new light by scrutinising them closely (again, what in poetry is called *ekphrasis* and in medicine close noticing). But this is not just sensate noticing; it is also a witnessing of suffering and of the human condition. Wallace Stevens (1951: 31) said that poetry doesn't reveal things, but instead lurks in material things where the world of poetry is "indistinguishable from the world in which we live". Normally, we don't see the world in the direct and intense way that poetry demands. It is up to poets to master the element of surprise to capture the intrinsic expressions of objects that count as revelations. For poetry, there is a formal set of heuristics and devices – such as verse forms, rhythm, cadence, assonance, consonance, dissonance, musicality and syncopation, intensity, density, alliteration, enjambment, rhyme, and repetition – that underpin the making of verse. These can be paralleled with Narrative Medicine's formal methods detailed by Charon such as use of plot, character, and metaphor.

Poetic work will encompass the patient's world, entering the rhythm of the heart, the immediate predictive arc of anticipation or what is to come, the anxiety and uncertainty embedded in the situation, a sense of awe and wonder at the body's diction, an efficiency of practiced intervention, and a moving dialogue with the patient that embodies care and instils confidence. William Carlos Williams (1967: 361, 362) cherishes the exchange of words between doctor and patient as necessarily poetic. What else could they be? Otherwise, they are brute, senseless:

> We begin to see that the underlying meaning of all they want to tell us and have always failed to communicate is the poem, the poem which their lives are being lived to realize. No one will believe it. And it is the actual words, as we hear them spoken under all circumstances, which contain it.

The medical work, for Williams, is "to recover underlying meaning as realistically as we recover metal out of ore". The poem is in the patient's words, where the poetic imagination is served by close noticing and witnessing, so that the patient is observed in exquisite detail, while idiosyncrasies are registered – not in objectification but in particularisation. Much of these offered riches are provided by traditional narrative medicine pedagogy. But like so much else in life, it matters how you get there, as the form of extraction and recovery of the precious metal. Poetry goes a different way from narrative. Perhaps it is a way you need. Perhaps it is a way you prefer. And perhaps it also gets to different places at different times, for a one-size-fits-all method is – distressingly – redolent of the biomedical. In summary, poetry can do things narrative cannot, and with panache, grace, and beauty; sometimes with wisdom too. And sometimes it will upset you or shift your perspective radically. The medical humanities can be seen as forms of poetry where they create intensity, diversity, and complexity out of the mundane. In short, the medical humanities can act as therapeutic media addressing medicine and medical education's symptoms. That is the mission. The process is by increasing the innovative metaphor count, and by transforming instrumental and economic biomedicine into an aesthetic, ethical, political, and spiritual practice.

Beckett redux

What we have set out to do in these two closing chapters is an incisive critical account of current approaches to narrative-based medicine within a historical context. In the process we have sprung poetry from its narrative prison. We have focused on Rita Charon's model of Narrative Medicine because of its reach and influence, and in the face of a lack of critical attention to its claims. We recognise huge value and importance in Charon's work, with its high level of innovation and leadership. But we also see a gap in the literature where Narrative Medicine has been treated descriptively rather than critically. We have our own plot in these two closing chapters – as developing a view of Narrative Medicine as an unacknowledged imperialistic device.

Have we unfairly caricatured generic narrative medicine and its commercial apogee in Narrative Medicine™? Readers can decide. From our roost in poetry pulpit, we recall Samuel Beckett's comparison of his own work with that of James Joyce from an interview in the *New York Times* (Shenker 1956): "He's tending towards omniscience and omnipotence as an artist. I'm working with impotence, ignorance". We leave "knowing" to narrative medicine as we proudly side with impotence and ignorance, defamiliarising clinical encounters so that they are made strange, comprised in ambiguity, and recognised as such. Here, we trudge in what Donald Schön (1984) famously called the "swampy lowlands" of values conflict rather than the "high, hard ground" of certainties.

Acknowledgement

This chapter was written in collaboration with Dr Shane Neilson.

REFERENCES

Abdel-Halim RE, AlKattan KM. Introducing medical humanities in the medical curriculum in Saudi Arabia: A pedagogical experiment. *Urology Annals*. 2012; 4: 73–79.

Adorno TW, Frenkel-Brunswik E, Levinson DJ, Sanford RN. 1950. *The Authoritarian Personality*. New York, NY: Harper and Row.

Agamben G. 1995. *Homo Sacer: Sovereign Power and Bare Life*. Palo Alto, CA: Stanford University Press.

Alduy C. (Undated). Against Narratives III. Or a Certain Kind of Narrative. Blog. Arcade: Literature, the Humanities & the World. Available at: http://www.arcade.stanford.edu/blogs/against-narratives-iii-or-certain-kind-narrative. Last accessed: 16/12/2022.

Allard J, Bleakley A, Hobbs A, Vinnell T. "Who's on the team today?" Collaborative teamwork in operating theatres should include briefing. *Journal of Interprofessional Care*. 2007; 21: 189–206.

Allard J, Bleakley A, Hobbs A, Coombes L. Pre-surgery briefings and safety climate in the operating theatre. *BMJ Quality and Safety*. 2011; 20: 711–17.

Arnaldi M. 2022. The translational imagination. In: A Bleakley, S Neilson (eds.) *Poetry in the Clinic: Towards a Lyrical Medicine*. Abingdon: Routledge, pp.270–72.

Baruch J. 2022. *Tornado of Life: A Doctor's Journey Through Constraints and Creativity in the ER*. Cambridge, MA: The MIT Press.

Barusch AS. *Refining the Narrative Turn: When does story-telling become research?* Gerontological Society of America. Nov. 16th 2012, San Diego, CA.

Bates V, Bleakley A, Goodman S. 2014. *Medicine, Health and the Arts: Approaches to the Medical Humanities*. Abingdon: Routledge.

Bates V, Hurwitz B. 2016. The roots and ramifications of narrative in modern medicine. In: A Whitehead, A Woods (eds.) *The Edinburgh Companion to the Critical Medical Humanities*. Edinburgh: Edinburgh University Press, pp.559–76.

Baudrillard J. 1983. *Simulations*. New York, NY: Semiotext(e).

Becker HS, Geer B, Hughes EC. 1961. *Boys in White*. New Jersey, NJ: Transaction Publishers.

Beckett S. 1953. *The Unnamable*. London: Faber & Faber.

Beckett S. 1966. Ping. Available at: www.https://samuelbeckett.blogspot.com/2012/01/ping-1966.html. Last accessed: 16/12/2022.

Berlin L. 2015. *A Manual for Cleaning Women*. London: Picador.

Bhabha H. 2004. *The Location of Culture*. London: Routledge.

Bishop JP. Rejecting medical humanism: Medical humanities and the metaphysics of medicine. *The Journal of Medical Humanities*. 2008; 29: 15–25.

Bleakley A. From reflective practice to holistic reflexivity. *Studies in Higher Education*. 1999; 24: 315–30.

Bleakley A. Stories as data, data as stories: Making sense of narrative inquiry in clinical education. *Medical Education*. 2005; 39: 534–40.

Bleakley A. Broadening conceptions of learning in medical education: The message from teamworking. *Medical Education*. 2006; 40: 150–57.

Bleakley A. Blunting Occam's razor: Aligning medical education with studies of complexity. *Journal of Evaluation in Clinical Practice*. 2010; 16: 849–55.

Bleakley A. Working in "Teams" in an Era of "Liquid" Healthcare: What is the use of theory? *Journal of Interprofessional Care*. 2013; 27: 18–26.

Bleakley A. 2014. *Patient-Centred Medicine in Transition: The Heart of the Matter*. Dordrecht: Springer.

Bleakley A. 2015. *The Medical Humanities and Medical Education: How the Medical Humanities Can Shape Better Doctors*. Abingdon: Routledge.

Bleakley A. Bargaining with Hypnos: Sleep deprivation in junior doctors as durational misperformance. *Performance Research*. 2016; 21: 49–52.

Bleakley A. 2017. *Thinking with Metaphors in Medicine: The State of the Art*. Abingdon: Routledge.

Bleakley A. Invoking the medical humanities to develop a #MedicineWeCanTrust. *Academic Medicine*. 2019; 10: 1422–24.

Bleakley A (ed). 2020a. *Routledge Handbook of the Medical Humanities*. Abingdon: Routledge.

Bleakley A. 2020b. *Educating Doctors Senses Through the Medical Humanities: "How Do I Look?"* Abingdon: Routledge.

Bleakley A. 2021. *Medical Education, Politics and Social Justice: The Contradiction Cure*. Abingdon: Routledge.

Bleakley A, Allard J, Hobbs A. 'Achieving ensemble': Communication in orthopaedic surgical teams and the development of situational awareness. *Advances in Health Sciences Education: Theory and Practice*. 2013; 18: 33–56.

Bleakley A, Bligh J, Browne J. 2011. *Medical Education for the Future: Identity, Power and Location*. Dordrecht: Springer.

Bleakley A, Brennan N. Does undergraduate curriculum design make a difference to readiness to practice as a junior doctor? *Medical Teacher*. 2011; 33: 459–67.

Bleakley A, Hobbs A, Boyden J, Walsh L. Safety in operating theatres: Improving teamwork through team resource management. *Journal of Workplace Learning*. 2004; 16: 83–91.

Bleakley A, Marshall R, Broemer R. Toward an aesthetic medicine: Developing a core medical humanities undergraduate curriculum. *Journal of Medical Humanities*. 2006; 27: 197–213.

Bleakley A, Neilson S. 2021. *Poetry in the Clinic: Towards a Lyrical Medicine*. Abingdon: Routledge.

Bleakley A, Neilson S. 2024. *The Routledge Handbook of Medicine and Poetry*. Abingdon: Routledge.

Boal A. 1991 (2nd ed.) *Theatre of the Oppressed*. London: Pluto Press.

Boothroyd D. 2000. Deconstruction and drugs: A philosophical/literary cocktail. In: N Royle (ed.) *Deconstructions: A User's Guide*. Basingstoke: Palgrave, pp.44–63.

Borrill C, West MA, Shapiro D, Rees A. Team working and effectiveness in health care. *British Journal of Health Care Management*. 2013; 6: 364–71.

Boseley S. 2006. 'Ritalin heart attacks warning urged after 51 deaths in US', *The Guardian*, 11 February. Available at: http://www.guardian.co.uk/frontpage/story/0,1707535,00. html. Last accessed: 16/12/2022.

Bourdieu P. 1977. *Outline of a Theory of Practice*. Cambridge: Cambridge University Press.

Bourke J. 2014. *The Story of Pain: From Prayer to Painkillers*. Oxford: Oxford University Press.

Brainard J, Hunter PR. Do complexity-informed health interventions work? A scoping review. *Implementation Science*. 2016; 11: 127.

Brennan N, Corrigan O, Allard J, et al. The transition from medical student to junior doctor: Today's experiences of Tomorrow's Doctors. *Medical Education*. 2010; 44: 449–58.

Brody H. My story is broken: Can you help me fix it? *Literature & Medicine*. 1994; 13: 91–94.

Bromiley M. 2015. Just a Routine Operation. Available at: https://www.youtube.com/ watch?v=JzlvgtPIof4. Last accessed: 16/12/2022.

Brook P. Emotional labour and the living personality at work: Labour power, materialist subjectivity and the dialogical self. *Culture and Organization*. 2013; 19: 332–52.

Brook P. 2022. *Seduced by Story: The Use and Abuse of Narrative*. New York, NY: New York Review Book.

Bruner J. 1986. *Actual Minds, Possible Worlds*. Cambridge, MA: Harvard University Press.

Bruner J. 2004. *Making Stories: Law, Literature, Life*. New York, NY: Farrar, Strauss & Giroux.

Byrne P, Long B. 1976. *Doctors Talking to Patients*. London: HMSO.

Campbell D. 2022. GPs giving antidepressants to children against guidelines. *The Guardian*, Friday 4th November 2022, p.5. Available at: https://www.theguardian.com/ society/2022/nov/04/gps-giving-antidepressants-to-children-against-guidelines. Last accessed: 17/12/2022.

Candido FJ, Souza R, Stumpf MA, et al. The use of drugs and medical students: A literature review. *Rev Assoc Med Bras*. 2018; 64: 462–68.

Canguilhem G. 1989. *The Normal and the Pathological*. New York, NY: Zone Books.

Capra F, Luisi PL. 2014. *The Systems View of Life: A Unifying Vision*. Cambridge: Cambridge University Press.

Casey E. 2013. *The Fate of Place: A Philosophical History*. Oakland, CA: University of California Press.

Centor RM. To be a great physician, you must understand the whole story. *Med Gen Med*. 2007; 9: 59.

Chambers T. 1999. *The Fiction of Bioethics: Cases as Literary Texts*. London: Routledge.

Chandler J, Rycroft-Malone J, Hawkes C, Noyes J. Application of simplified Complexity Theory concepts for healthcare social systems to explain the implementation of evidence into practice. *Journal of Advanced Nursing*. 2015; 72: 461–80.

Charon R. Narrative medicine: A model for empathy, reflection, profession, and trust. *Journal of the American Medical Association*. 2001; 286: 1897–902.

Charon R. 2006. *Narrative Medicine: Honoring the Stories of Illness*. Oxford: Oxford University Press.

Charon R, Montello M (eds.) 2002. *Stories Matter: The Role of Narrative in Medical Ethics*. London: Routledge.

Charon R, Wyer P. Narrative evidence based medicine. *Lancet*. 2008; 26: 296–97.

Charon R, DasGupta S, Hermann N, et al. 2016. *The Principles and Practices of Narrative Medicine.* Oxford: Oxford University Press.

Cristancho S, Field E, Lingard L. What is the state of complexity science in medical education research? *Medical Education.* 2019; 53: 95–104.

Cleland J, Walker K, Gale M, Nicol LJ. Simulation-based education: Understanding the complexity of a surgical training 'Boot Camp'. *Medical Education.* 2016; 50: 829–41.

Cole TR, Carlin NS, Carson R. 2015. *Medical Humanities.* Cambridge: Cambridge University Press.

Colón-Ramos DA. The need to connect: On the cell biology of synapses, behaviors, and networks in science. *Mol Biol Cell.* 2016; 27: 3197–201.

Cooper N, Frain J. 2017. *ABC of Clinical Communication.* Chichester: Wiley Blackwell.

Crawford P, Brown B, Tischler V, Baker C. Health humanities: The future of medical humanities? *Mental Health Review Journal.* 2010; 15: 4–10.

Crawford P, Brown B, Baker C, et al. 2015. *Health Humanities.* Basingstoke: Palgrave Macmillan.

Crawford P, Brown B, Charise A. 2020. *The Routledge Companion to Health Humanities.* Abingdon: Routledge.

Cristancho S, Field E, Lingard L. What is the state of complexity science in medical education research? *Medical Education.* 2019; 53: 95–104.

Deleuze G, Guattari F. 2004a, b. *A Thousand Plateaus* (2 vols). London: Continuum.

Derrida J. The rhetoric of drugs. An interview. *Differences.* 1993; 5: 1–25.

Doctorow EL. 1976. *Ragtime.* London: Macmillan.

Dolan B. 2015. *Humanitas: Readings in the Development of the Medical Humanities.* San Francisco, CA: University of California Medical Humanities Press.

Doll W, Fleener MJ, Trueit D, St Julien J. 2005. *Chaos, Complexity, Curriculum, and Culture: A Conversation.* New York, NY: Peter Lang.

Dyre L, Gierson L, Rasmussen KMB, et al. The concept of errors in medical education: A scoping review. *Advances in Health Sciences Education.* 2022; 27: 761–92.

Duvefelt H. Listen to your patient's story: It's their diagnosis. Hans Duvefelt MD/ Physician. December 14, 2016. Available at: https://www.kevinmd.com/blog/2016/12/listen-patients-story-diagnosis.html. Last accessed: 16/12/2022.

Eagleton T. 1983. *Literary Theory: An Introduction.* Minneapolis, MN: University of Minneapolis Press.

Eichbaum Q, Barbeau-Meunier C-A, White M, et al. Empathy across cultures - one size does not fit all: From ego-logical to the eco-logical of relational empathy. *Advances in Health Sciences Education Theory & Practice.* 2022; 28: 643–57.

Eliot TS. 1934. *The Rock.* London: Harcourt, Brace & Co.

Ellis BE. 2005. *Lunar Park.* London: Picador.

Engeström Y. 2008. *From Teams to Knots: Activity-Theoretical Studies of Collaboration and Learning at Work.* Cambridge: Cambridge University Press.

Engeström Y. 2018. *Expertise in Transition: Expansive Learning in Medical Work.* Cambridge: Cambridge University Press.

Evans HM, Greaves DA. Developing the medical humanities–report of a research colloquium, and collected abstracts of papers. *Medical Humanities.* 2001a; 27: 93–98.

Evans HM, Greaves DA. Medical humanities at the University of Wales Swansea. *Medical Humanities.* 2001b; 27: 51–52.

Evans HM, Greaves DA. "Medical Humanities" – What's in a Name? *Medical Humanities.* 2002; 28: 1–2.

Fenwick T, Dahlgren MA. Towards socio-material approaches in simulation-based education: Lessons from complexity theory. *Medical Education.* 2015; 49: 359–67.

Fieschi L, Matarese M, Vellone E. Medical humanities in healthcare education in Italy: A literature review. *Annali dell'Istituto Superiore di Sanità.* 2013; 49: 56–64.

Foucault M. 1970. *The Order of Things: An Archaeology of the Human Sciences.* London: Tavistock Publications.

Foucault M. 1976. *The Birth of the Clinic: An Archaeology of Medical Perception.* London: Routledge.

Foucault M. 1991. *Discipline and Punish: The Birth of the Prison.* Harmondsworth: Penguin.

Foucault M. 2005. The *Hermeneutics of the Subject: Lectures at the Collège de France 1981–1982.* New York, NY: Picador.

Foucault M. 2006. *The History of Madness.* Abingdon: Routledge.

Foucault M. 2020. *Power.* London: Penguin.

Frambach J, Driessen EW, van der Vleuten CPM. Using activity theory to study cultural complexity in medical education. *Perspectives on Medical Education.* 2014; 3: 190–203.

Frank AW. 1995. *The Wounded Storyteller: Body, Illness and Ethics.* Chicago, IL: University of Chicago Press.

Franzen J. 2001. *The Corrections.* London: Fourth Estate.

Freire P. 1996. *Pedagogy of the Oppressed.* Harmondsworth: Penguin.

Freud S, Breuer J. 2004. *Studies in Hysteria.* London: Penguin.

Gabbay J, le May A. Mindlines: Making sense of evidence in practice. *British Journal of General Practice.* 2016; 66: 402–03.

Geddes L. 2022. DeepMind uncovers structure of 200m proteins in scientific leap forward. *The Guardian,* 28 Jul 2022. Available at: https://www.theguardian.com/technology/2022/jul/28/deepmind-uncovers-structure-of-200m-proteins-in-scientific-leap-forward. Last accessed: 17/12/2022.

Geertz C. 1973. *The Interpretation of Cultures.* New York, NY: Basic Books.

Geller G, Grbic D, Andolsek KM, et al. Tolerance for ambiguity amongst medical students: Patterns of change during medical school and their implications for professional development. *Academic Medicine.* 2021; 96: 1036–42.

General Medical Council (GMC). 1993. *Tomorrow's Doctors.* London: GMC.

General Medical Council (GMC). 2003. *Tomorrow's Doctors: Recommendations on Undergraduate Medical Education.* London: GMC.

Gill A, Nelson EA, Mian A, et al. Responding to moderate breaches in professionalism: An intervention for medical students. *Medical Teacher.* 2015; 37: 136–39.

Glouberman S, Zimmerman B. 2002. Complicated and Complex Systems: What Would Successful Reform of Medicare Look Like? Commission on the Future of Healthcare in Canada: Discussion Paper 8. Available at: https://www.alnap.org/system/files/content/resource/files/main/complicatedandcomplexsystems-zimmermanreport-medicare-reform.pdf. Last accessed: 17/12/2022.

Goffman E. 1990. *The Presentation of Self in Everyday Life.* London: Penguin Books.

Goldenberg I, Matheson K, Mantler J. The assessment of emotional intelligence: A comparison of performance-based and self-report methodologies. *Journal of Personality Assessment.* 2006; 86: 33–45.

Goodman P. 1966. *Compulsory Miseducation and the Community of Scholars.* London: Random House.

Goodwin B. 1994. *How the Leopard Changed its Spots: The Evolution of Complexity.* New York, NY: Touchstone.

Gorz A. 2010. *The Immaterial.* London: Seagull Books.

Grassberger P. Towards a quantitative theory of self-generated complexity. *International Journal of Theoretical Physics.* 1986; 25: 907–38.

Green B, Oeppen RS, Smith DW, Brennan PA. Challenging hierarchy in healthcare teams – ways to flatten gradients to improve teamwork and patient care. *British Journal of Oral and Maxillofacial Surgery.* 2017; 55: 449–53.

Greene R (ed.) 2012 (4th ed.) *The Princeton Encyclopaedia of Poetry & Poetics.* Princeton, NJ: Princeton University Press.

Greenhalgh T, Hurwitz B (eds.) 1998. *Narrative Based Medicine: Dialogue and Discourse in Clinical Practice.* London: BMJ Books.

Greenhalgh T, Hurwitz B. Narrative based medicine: Why study narrative? *British Medical Journal.* 1999; 318: 48–50.

Grugulis I, Warhurst C, Keep E. 2004. What's happening to skill? In: C Warhurst, I Grugulis, E Keep (eds.). *The Skills that Matter.* Basingstoke: Palgrave MacMillan.

Gutkind L (ed.) 2007. *Silence Kills: Speaking Out and Saving Lives.* Dallas, TX: Southern Methodist University Press.

Guyatt G, Cairns J, Churchill D, et al. Evidence-based medicine: A new approach to teaching the practice of medicine. *Journal of the American Medical Association.* 1992; 268: 2420–25.

Han PK, Schupack D, Daggett S, et al. Temporal changes in tolerance of uncertainty among medical students: insights from an exploratory study. *Medical Education Online.* 2015; 20: 28285.

Hancock J, Mattick K. Tolerance of ambiguity and psychological well-being in medical training: A systematic review. *Medical Education.* 2020; 54: 125–37.

Hardt M, Negri A. 2000. *Empire.* Cambridge, MA: Harvard University Press.

Hardt M, Negri A. 2006. *Multitude.: War and Democracy in the Age of Empire.* London: Penguin.

Hardt M, Negri A. 2009. *Commonwealth.* Cambridge, MA: Harvard University Press.

Hardt M, Negri A. 2017. *Assembly.* Oxford: Oxford University Press.

Harman G. 2018. *Object-Oriented Ontology: A New Theory of Everything.* London: Pelican.

Haslam D. 2022. *Side Effects: How Our Healthcare Lost its Way and How We Fix It.* London: Atlantic Books.

Heron J. 1977. *Dimensions of Facilitator Style.* London: British Postgraduate Medical Federation.

Heron J. 2001 (5th ed.) *Helping the Client: A Creative, Practical Guide.* London: Sage.

Hill A. 1945. *Art versus Illness: A Story of Art Therapy.* London: Allen & Unwin.

Hillman J. 1980. *Egalitarian Typologies Versus the Perception of the Unique.* Dallas, TX: Spring Publications.

Hochschild AR. 1983. *The Managed Heart: Commercialization of Human Feeling.* Berkeley, CA: University of California Press.

Hooker C, Noonan E. Medical humanities as expressive of western culture. *Medical Humanities.* 2011; 37: 79–84.

Hunley S. Can Hallucinogens Treat Anxiety and Depression? Available at: https://www.anxiety.org/lsd-hallucinogenic-mushrooms-to-treat-anxiety-and-depression. Last accessed: 18/12/2022.

Hunter KM. 1991. *Doctors' Stories: The Narrative Structure of Medical Knowledge.* Princeton, NJ: Princeton University Press.

Hyvärinen M. 2012. *"Against Narrativity" Reconsidered.* Bern: Peter Lang.

James EC. 2010. Global Health and Medical Humanities. Available at: https://www.betterworld.mit.edu/global-health-and-medical-humanities/. Last accessed: 18/12/2022.

John M. From Osler to the cone technique. *HSRC Proc Intensive Care Cardiovascular Anesthetics.* 2013; 5: 57–58.

Jones EM, Tansey EM (eds.) 2015. *The Development of Narrative Practices in Medicine c.1960-c.2000.* Wellcome Witnesses to Contemporary Medicine. Vol. 52. London: Queen Mary University of London.

Jones T, Wear D, Freidman L (eds.) 2014. *Health Humanities Reader.* New Jersey, NJ: Rutgers University Press.

Jorm C, Nisbet G, Roberts C, et al. Using complexity theory to develop a student-directed interprofessional learning activity for 1220 healthcare students. *BMC Medical Education.* 2016; 16: 199.

Jorm C, Roberts C. Using complexity theory to guide medical school evaluations. *Academic Medicine.* 2018; 93: 399–405.

Kaiser R. Fixing identity by denying uniqueness: An analysis of professional identity in medicine. *Journal of Medical Humanities.* 2002; 23: 95–102.

Kalanithi P. 2016. *When Breath Becomes Air.* London: Bodley Head.

Kant I. 1784/1996. *An Answer to the Question: What is Enlightenment?* In: J Schmidt (ed.) 1996. *What is Enlightenment? Eighteenth-Century Answers and Twentieth-Century Questions.* Berkeley, CA: University of California Press, pp.58–64.

Kauffman S. 1995. *At Home in the Universe: The Search for the Laws of Self-Organisation and Complexity.* London: Viking.

Kidd MJ, Connor JT. Striving to do good things: Teaching humanities in Canadian Medical Schools. *Journal of Medical Humanities.* 2008; 29: 45–54.

Kleinman A. 1988. *The Illness Narratives.* New York: Basic Books.

Kleinsinger F. Working with the noncompliant patient. *The Permanente Journal.* 2010; 14: 54.

Kristeva J. 1982. *Approaching Abjection: Powers of Horror.* New York, NY: Columbia University Press.

Kristeva J, Moro M-R, Odemark J, Engebretsen E. 2020. The cultural crossings of care: A call for translational medical humanities. In: A Bleakley (ed.) *Routledge Handbook of the Medical Humanities.* Abingdon: Routledge.

Lacquer T. 1989. *Making Sex: Body and Gender from the Greeks to Freud.* Cambridge, MA: Harvard University Press.

Launer J. 2002. *Narrative-Based Primary Care. A Practical Guide.* Abington, UK: Radcliffe Medical Press.

Law J. 2006. *Big Pharma: How the World's Biggest Drug Companies Control Illness.* London: Constable.

Levine D, Bleakley A. Maximising medicine through aphorisms. *Medical Education.* 2012; 46: 153–62.

Lefève C, Thoreau F, Zimmer A (eds.) 2020. *Les humanités médicales: L'engagement des sciences humaines et sociales en médecine (La personne en médecine).* Paris: Institut La Personne en medicine.

Lewis T. 2012. *The Aesthetics of Education: Theatre, Curiosity, and Politics in the work of Jacques Rancière and Paulo Freire.* London: Bloomsbury.

Lingard L, McDougall A, Levstik M, et al. Representing complexity well: A story about teamwork, with implications for how we teach collaboration. *Medical Education.* 2012; 46: 869–77.

Lorenz E. Deterministic non-periodic flow. *Journal of the Atmospheric Sciences.* 1963; 20: 130–41.

Lyotard J-F. 1979. *The Postmodern Condition: A Report on Knowledge.* Manchester: Manchester University Press.

Macdonald CL, Sirianni C. 1996. The service society and the changing experience of work. In: CL Macdonald, C Sirianni (eds.) *On Working in the Service Society.* Philadelphia, PA: Temple University Press, pp.1–28.

Macneill P (ed.) 2014. *Ethics and the Arts*. Dordrecht: Springer.

Mangione S, Chakraborti C, Staltari G, et al. Medical students' exposure to the humanities correlates with positive personal qualities and reduced burnout: A multi-institutional U.S. Survey. *Journal of General Internal Medicine*. 2018; 33: 628–34.

McGough JJ, Pataki CS, Suddath R. Dexmethylphenidate extended-release capsules for attention deficit hyperactivity disorder. *Expert Review of Neurotherapeutics*. 2004; 9: 437–41.

Mennin, S. Self-organisation, integration and curriculum in the complex world of medical education. *Medical Education*. 2010; 44: 20–30.

Miéville C. 2009. *The City & The City*. London: Picador Classic.

Mol A-M. 2002. *The Body Multiple: Ontology in Medical Practice*. Durham, NC: Duke University Press.

Montgomery K. 2006. *How Doctors Think: Clinical Judgement and the Practice of Medicine*. Oxford: Oxford University Press.

Monrouxe L, Rees C, Dennis I, et al. Professionalism dilemmas, moral distress and the healthcare student: Insights from two online UK-wide questionnaire studies. *BMJ Open*. 2014; 5: e007518.

Montgomery K. 2006. *How Doctors Think: Clinical Judgment and the Practice of Medicine*. New York, NY: Oxford University Press.

Montello M (ed.) 2014. *Narrative Ethics: The Role of Stories in Bioethics*. The Hastings Center Report Vol. 44, Issue S1, Jan-Feb 2014, pp.S2–6.

Moody R. 2002. *The Black Veil*. London: Faber & Faber.

Moody N, Hallam J (eds.) 1998. *Medical Fictions*. Liverpool: The John Moores University.

Mukherjee S. 2022. *The Song of the Cell: An Exploration of Medicine and the New Human*. London: The Bodley Head.

Neilson S. A logical development: Biomedicine's fingerprints are on the instrument of close reading in Charonian Narrative Medicine. *Medical Humanities*. 2022; 48: e9.

O'Mahony S. Against narrative medicine. *Perspectives in Biology and Medicine*. 2013; 56: 611–19.

O'Neill D. Surprised by Beauty. June 19, 2015. Available at: https://www.stg-blogs.bmj.com/bmj/2015/06/19/desmond-oneill-surprised-by-beauty/. Last accessed: 18/12/2022.

Ospina NS, Phillips KA, Rodriguez-Gutierrez R, et al. Eliciting the patient's agenda- secondary analysis of recorded clinical encounters. *Journal of General Internal Medicine*. 2018; 34: 36–40.

Peterkin A, Bleakley A. 2017. *Staying Human During the Foundation Programme and Beyond: How to Thrive After Medical School*. Baton Rouge, FL: CRC Press.

Peterkin A, Skorzewska A. 2018. *Health Humanities in Postgraduate Medical Education*. Oxford: OUP.

Peterkin A, Beausoleil N, Kidd M, et al. 2020. Medical humanities in Canadian medical schools: Progress, challenges and opportunities. In A Bleakley (ed.) *Routledge Handbook of the Medical Humanities*. Abingdon: Routledge, pp.364–80.

Petersen A, Bleakley A, Broemer R, Marshall R. The medical humanities today: Humane healthcare or tool of governance? *Journal of Medical Humanities*. 2008; 29: 1–4.

Pinar WF, Reynolds WM, Slattery P, Taubman PM (eds.) 1995. *Understanding Curriculum: An Introduction to the Study of Historical and Contemporary Curriculum Discourses*. New York, NY: Peter Lang.

Pinar WF. 2004. *What is Curriculum Theory?* Mahwah, NJ: Lawrence Erlbaum.

Pinar WF. 2019 (3rd ed.) *What is Curriculum Theory?* New York, NY: Routledge.

Pinsky, M. Complexity modeling: Identify instability early. *Critical Care Medicine*. 2010; 30: S649–55.

Plsek P, Greenhalgh T. The challenge of complexity in healthcare. *British Medical Journal.* 2001; 323: 625–28.

Plsek P, Sweeney K, Griffiths F. 2002. *Complexity and Healthcare: An Introduction.* Oxford: Radcliffe.

Portmann A. 1967. *Animal Forms and Patterns: A Study of the Appearance of Animals.* New York, NY: Schocken Books.

Pound P, Britten N, Morgan M, et al. Resisting medicines: A synthesis of qualitative studies of medicine taking. *Social Science & Medicine.* 2005; 61: 133–55.

Prideaux S. 2018. *I am Dynamite!: A Life of Friedrich Nietzsche.* London: Faber & Faber.

Propp V. 1968: *Morphology of the Folktale.* Austin, TX: University of Texas Press.

Ramaswamy R, Ramaswamy R. 2020. Desire imagination action: Theatre of the Oppressed in medical education. In: A Bleakley (ed.) *Routledge Handbook of Medical Humanities.* 2020, pp.250–56.

Rancière J. 1991. *The Ignorant Schoolmaster: Five Lessons in Intellectual Emancipation.* Stanford, CA: Stanford University Press.

Rancière J. 1995. *On the Shores of Politics.* London: Verso.

Rancière J. 2006a. *Hatred of Democracy.* London: Verso.

Rancière J. 2006b. *The Politics of Aesthetics.* New York: Continuum.

Rancière J. 2010. *Dissensus: On Politics and Aesthetics.* London: Continuum.

Rancière J. 2011. *The Emancipated Spectator.* London: Verso.

Rancière J. 2013. *Aisthesis: Scenes from the Aesthetic Regime of Art.* London: Verso.

Randerson J. *The Independent.* Mon 8 Dec. *Revealed: child labour used to make NHS instruments.* Available at: https://www.theguardian.com/society/2008/dec/08/nhs-instruments-child-labour. Last accessed: 18/12/2022.

Richtel M. This Teen Was Prescribed 10 Psychiatric Drugs. She's Not Alone. *The New York Times*, 27 Aug. 2022 (updated Dec 14 2022). Available at: https://www.nytimes.com/2022/08/27/health/teens-psychiatric-drugs.html. Last accessed: 18/12/2022.

Rilke R-M. 2013. *Letters to a Young Poet.* Scotts Valley, CA: CreateSpace Independent Publishing Platform.

Rose N. 2007. *The Politics of Life Itself.* Princeton, NJ: Princeton University Press.

Ross S, Maxwell S. Prescribing and the core curriculum for tomorrow's doctors: BPS curriculum in clinical pharmacology and prescribing for medical students. *British Journal of Clinical Pharmacology.* 2012; 74: 644–61.

Sabbagh D. 2022. Ukrainians use phone app to spot deadly Russian drone attacks. *The Guardian,* Sat. 29 Oct 2022. Available at: https://www.theguardian.com/world/2022/oct/29/ukraine-phone-app-russia-drone-attacks-eppo. Last accessed: 18/12/2022.

Salehi P. 2016. Hierarchy in Medicine: Compromising Values for Honors. Available at: https://www.in-training.org/hierarchy-medicine-compromising-values-honors-11362. Last accessed: 18/12/2022.

Said E. 1978. *Orientalism.* New York, NY: Pantheon Books.

Sartre J-P. 2003. *Being and Nothingness: An Essay on Phenomenological Ontology.* Abingdon: Routledge.

Sartwell C. 2000. *End of Story: Towards an Annihilation of Language and History.* Albany, NY: State University of New York Press.

Schleifer R, Vannatta JB. 2013. *The Chief Concern of Medicine: The Integration of the Medical Humanities and Narrative Knowledge into Medical Practices.* Ann Arbor, MI: University of Michigan Press.

Schmidt J (ed.) 1996. *What is Enlightenment? Eighteenth-Century Answers and Twentieth-Century Questions.* Berkeley, CA: University of California Press.

Schön D. 1984. *The Reflective Practitioner*. New York, NY: Basic Books.

Shaw MK, Rees CE, Andersen NB, et al. Professionalism lapses and hierarchies: A qualitative analysis of medical students' narrated acts of resistance. *Social Science & Medicine*. 2018; 219: 45–53.

Shenker I. MOODY MAN OF LETTERS; A Portrait of Samuel Beckett, Author of the Puzzling 'Waiting For Godot'. *New York Times*, May 6, 1956. Available at: https://www.nytimes.com/1956/05/06/archives/moody-man-of-letters-a-portrait-of-samuel-beckett-author-of-the.html. Last accessed: 18/12/2022.

Shklovsky V. 1991. *Theory of Prose*. London: Dalkey Archive Press.

Singh R, Pushkin GW. How should medical education better prepare physicians for opioid prescribing? *American Medical Association Journal of Ethics*. 2019; 21: E636–641.

Slouka N. 2010. *Essays from the Nick of Time: Reflections and Refutations*. Minneapolis, MN: Graywolf Press.

Steiner P. 1984. *Russian Formalism: A Metapoetics*. Ithaca, NY: Cornell University Press.

Stevens W. 1951. *The Necessary Angel*. London: Knopf.

Strawson G. Against narrativity. *Ratio*. 2004a; 17: 428–52.

Strawson G. 2004b. Tales of the unexpected. *The Guardian*, Jan 10 2004. Available at: https://www.theguardian.com/books/2004/jan/10/society.philosophy. Last accessed: 19/12/2022.

Szalai J. How Reality Got 'Storified' and What We Can Do About It. *New York Times*, Oct 19 2022. Available at: https://www.nytimes.com/2022/10/19/books/review/seduced-by-story-peter-brooks.html. Last accessed: 18/12/2022.

Szalavitz M. 2022. The War on Drugs Has a Warning for Post-Roe America. *New York Times*, July 26, 2022. Available at: https://www.nytimes.com/2022/07/26/opinion/medicine-criminal-law.html. Last accessed: 19/12/2022.

Thomas C. 2005. Ellis Writes Himself into Suburbs. SF Gate: *San Francisco Chronicle*, 14 Aug 2005. Available at: https://www.sfgate.com/books/article/Ellis-writes-himself-into-suburbs-2647761.php. Last accessed: 19/12/2022.

Tickle L. Why does so much of the NHS's surgical equipment start life in the sweatshops of Pakistan? *The Independent*, Mon 19 January 2015. Available at: https://www.independent.co.uk/life-style/health-and-families/features/why-does-so-much-of-the-nhs-s-surgical-equipment-start-life-in-the-sweatshops-of-pakistan-9988885.html. Last accessed: 19/12/2022.

Trent R. 2019. What role does the science of complexity play in medicine? Available at: https://www.kevinmd.com/blog/2019/08/what-role-does-the-science-of-complexity-play-in-medicine.html.

Trueit D (ed.) 2013. *Pragmatism, Post-modernism, and Complexity Theory: The 'Fascinating Imaginative Realm' of William E. Doll, Jr*. London: Routledge.

Tuffin R. Implications of complexity theory for clinical practice and healthcare organization. *BJA Education*. 2016; 16: 349–52.

Vaihinger H. 1924. *The Philosophy of "As If"*. London: Routledge.

Van Dijck J. 2005. *The Transparent Body: A Cultural Analysis of Medical Imaging*. Seattle, WA: University of Washington Press.

Verghese A. 1995. *My Own Country: A Doctor's Story*. New York, NY: Simon & Schuster.

Verghese A. 1999. *The Tennis Partner*. London: Chatto & Windus.

Verghese A. 2009. *Cutting for Stone*. London: Chatto and Windus.

Verghese A. 2015. The physician as storyteller. In: B Dolan. *Humanitas: Readings in the Development of the Medical Humanities*. San Francisco, CA: University of California Medical Humanities Press, pp.224–35.

Wallace DF. 1996. *Infinite Jest*. London: Abacus.

Warhurst C, Nickson D. 2020. *Aesthetic Labour.* London: Sage.

Warmington S. 2020. *Storytelling Encounters as Medical Education: Crafting Relational Identity.* Abingdon: Routledge.

Weiss P. 2005. *The Aesthetics of Resistance Vol. I.* Durham, NC: Duke University Press.

Weiss P. 2020. *The Aesthetics of Resistance Vol. II.* Durham, NC: Duke University Press

West MA, Lyubovnikova J. Illusions of team working in health care. *Journal of Health Organization and Management.* 2013; 27: 134–42.

White H. 1987. *The Content of the Form: Narrative Discourse and Narrative Representation.* Baltimore, MD: The Johns Hopkins University Press.

Whitehead A, Woods A (eds.) 2016. *The Edinburgh Companion to the Critical Medical Humanities*. Edinburgh: Edinburgh University Press.

Wieringa S, Greenhalgh T. 10 years of mindlines: A systematic review and commentary. *Implementation Science.* 2015; 10: 45.

Williams WC. 1967. *The Autobiography of William Carlos Williams.* New York, NY: New Directions.

Wohlmann A. 2022. *Metaphor in Illness Writing: Fight and Battle Reused.* Edinburgh: Edinburgh University Press.

Woods A. The limits of narrative: Provocations for the medical humanities. *Medical Humanities.* 2011a; 37: 73–78.

Woods A. Post-narrative: An appeal. *Narrative Inquiry.* 2011b; 21: 399–406.

Wulf A. 2022. *Magnificent Rebels: The First Romantics and the Invention of the Self.* London: John Murray.

Yakubinski LP. 2018. *On Language and Poetry: Three Essays*. New York, NY: Upper West Side Philosophers Inc.

Zaharias G. Narrative-based medicine 1. *Canadian Family Physician.* 2018; 64: 176–80.

INDEX